Developing
a Healthcare
Research Proposal

For George

Maxine Offredy

For my family and my former and present research students
Peter Vickers

Developing a Healthcare Research Proposal:

An Interactive Student Guide

Maxine Offredy PhD
Reader in Primary Health Care
Centre for Research in Primary and Community Care
University of Hertfordshire
Hatfield
UK

Peter Vickers PhD
Visiting Research and Teaching Fellow
Faculty of Health and Human Science
University of Hertfordshire
Hatfield
UK

WILEY-BLACKWELL

A John Wiley & Sons, Ltd., Publication

Blackwell Publishing was acquired by John Wiley & Sons in February 2007. Blackwell's publishing programme has been merged with Wiley's global Scientific, Technical, and Medical business to form Wiley-Blackwell.

Registered office
John Wiley & Sons Ltd, The Atrium, Southern Gate, Chichester, West Sussex, PO19 8SQ, United Kingdom

Editorial office
9600 Garsington Road, Oxford, OX4 2DQ, United Kingdom
2121 State Avenue, Ames, Iowa 50014-8300, USA

For details of our global editorial offices, for customer services and for information about how to apply for permission to reuse the copyright material in this book please see our website at www.wiley.com/wiley-blackwell.

Library of Congress Cataloging-in-Publication Data

Offredy, Maxine.
   Developing a research proposal for healthcare professionals : an interactive research / Maxine Offredy, Peter Vickers.
        p. ; cm.
   Includes bibliographical references and index.
   ISBN 978-1-4051-8337-6 (pbk. : alk. paper) 1. Medicine–Research–
Methodology. 2. Allied health personnel. I. Vickers, Peter. II. Title.
   [DNLM: 1. Research–methods. 2. Data Collection–methods. 3. Research Design.
WA 20.5 O32d 2010]
   R852.O34 2010
   610.72–dc22

                                                                       2009035249

A catalogue record for this book is available from the British Library.

Set in 10/12pt Palatino by Toppan Best-set Premedia Limited

1 2010

Contents

On the Web: http://www.researchproposalsforhealthprofessionals.com

Preface

This book reflects our experiences as practitioners, research students and teachers of the topic. It is intended to be helpful to those who are novices to research and to provide a step-by-step approach to their understanding of some of the issues relating to evidence-based practice. We assume that readers have no knowledge of the subject and so we have tried to present the contents in a way that facilitates understanding and increases knowledge.

Most books attempting to explain the research process do so in an abstract, academic way. However, health professionals work in a very practical environment, and nursing students spend half of their education in the clinical/practical environment. As a consequence, health professionals often experience a gap between their own experiences and the relevance that they perceive research to be for them from the many academic/abstract books on research theory and methodology they may access. Both authors are engaged in clinical research, so, whilst not excluding or belittling the academic underpinning of research, research methodology and the research process, we have set the whole theoretical discipline of research within a much more practical milieu. This allows health professionals to understand what is meant by research and its importance to their own, 'real' world. By making research knowledge an integral part of healthcare, we hope to generate enthusiasm for the subject and improve patient care.

Introduction

You have decided that you want to undertake some research, but how do you go about it? This book and the accompanying web program will answer this question and will help you to start your research by introducing you to the concepts, theories and practical implications of undertaking a research study from start to finish, as well as helping you to write a research proposal – the first and most important part of your research study.

Many people – health professionals among them – have the wrong impression about research. They see it as something that can only be done by academics – people with very high IQs, who are remote from the real world, live in 'ivory towers' and who have been specially trained to do research. When you ask some people what researchers are like, you will often get descriptions of 'mad scientists' or Dr Frankenstein types – people continually interfering with nature. This could not be further from the truth. Most research is carried out by ordinary men and women who have a passion for their subject and want to find out more about it. In other words, people like you and me. As you will find out by reading this book, there are many types of research, and yes, some does take place in laboratories. However, much research takes place in ordinary settings – in hospitals, homes, on the street, and so on.

Reflection
Take a few minutes to think about some research that you have done recently.

How many of you reached the conclusion that you have never done any research? Probably most of you, unless you have undertaken an academic degree. But, in fact, you would be quite wrong. If you think about it, you have all undertaken some research, not just once or twice, but almost every day.

What is research?

Let us think again about what research is. All right, you may not have finished up with a written report illustrated with lots of graphs and tables, but you will certainly have undertaken research into something that is of interest to you. For example, how many of you own a car? How did you decide to buy that particular make and model? You compared different makes and models, different prices, differences in running costs, and so on. You probably talked to people who have similar cars and you may have road-tested different makes before coming to the conclusion that the car you bought was the one for you. If you did all or some of this, then you have done research, because this comparison, soliciting opinions and testing are all skills that we use in research. The only difference is that in 'real' research we go about the task in a more structured and scientific way – although there are people who choose their cars very scientifically.

> **To Do**
>
> Now you have seen one example of how you undertake research in everyday life, spend a few minutes thinking of other examples of everyday research similar to that one.

Here are a few examples:

- **Relationships** – when you first meet somebody, you spend some time observing and 'researching' them, for example, you talk to them in order to find out what they do for a living, their interests and hobbies, their beliefs and opinions, and other important facts about them, such as their sense of humour, physical attractiveness and whether they find you interesting and attractive.
- **Restaurants for a special evening out** – you may read reviews of restaurants in your area, or talk to friends and colleagues to find out where they would go for a celebration.

- **Where to go on holiday** – again, you probably read reviews in magazines of destinations, you talked to travel agents as well as friends and colleagues, you collected and compared brochures of places to visit, and you looked at the costs.
- **Buying things for the house** – for example, if you wish to buy a refrigerator, you will read reviews of different makes, you will talk to salespeople in a variety of shops/dealers and you will compare things such as size, running costs, effects on the environment and, of course, prices.
- **Banks/building societies for savings, investments and mortgages** – again, you will need to do some research so that you can compare interest rates, the efficiency and friendliness of the staff, ease of access, and these days, reliability and security.
- **Where to live** – before you decide where you want to live, you will need to do some research into the area, including the price of houses or the cost of renting accommodation, distance from your place of work or the availability of work in the area, schools (if you have children), the physical environment, entertainment venues/nightlife, restaurants and other facilities, crime rates and ease (or difficulty) of accessibility to family.

You can probably think of many more examples where you undertake research to help you in your daily life. So you can see that you are already 'researchers' because you are doing it all the time and have developed many of the skills necessary for more formal research.

Being a researcher

So what makes a researcher? Probably the three most important qualities are curiosity, passion and 'doggedness'. Why do we put these three at the head of the list of qualities that a researcher needs? Well, the reason is that these are the three qualities that a good researcher needs in order to identify something that they wish to look at in more detail (the research), and to know that this is what they wish to spend the next few months or even years doing.

Curiosity is essential because we need to be curious about the topic we wish to research. For example, why does this work but not that? What will the outcome be if I make this change? How can I improve the care of my patients? Which is the more effective, but cheaper, treatment? And so we can go on with the many questions that you must have asked yourself in the course of your work (you probably would not be reading this book if you had not asked yourself such questions). So, curiosity is often the starting point for any research project.

Turning now to passion, this is essential because if you are only half-hearted about what you want to research, then either you will get bored with it and abandon the research or, if you do manage to complete the research project, because you have not put all your effort into it, the result will be substandard.

Finally, the third most important quality of the researcher, doggedness, is important because of the length of time that a good research project will take from formulating the initial idea of doing the research to its completion, the writing up, dissemination of the findings and (hopefully) the implementation of your results, can almost take over your life. It is always easy to find something else that you would prefer to do.

Without the three qualities of curiosity, passion and doggedness, the research may well not be completed. To give a personal example, when one of the authors started his PhD as a part-time student, he was one of eight students who commenced around the same time. Of those eight, only two were interested in the topic that they wanted to research and were studying for a PhD because that would allow them to undertake the research with more guidance and academic rigour. The other six had decided that they wanted to do a PhD, and then looked for a subject that they could research. In other words, they had done the opposite to the other two. Of the eight who commenced their PhD studies at around the same time, after seven years' part-time study and research only two had completed their research and been awarded a PhD, and, as you probably guessed, the two who completed were the two with a curiosity and a passion for what they were researching, along with the doggedness to complete the research and write it up. To keep going for all the years that a research project can take, particularly if you are undertaking the research on your own rather than as part of a team, requires passion, curiosity and doggedness above all else.

Reflection

In addition to the three qualities discussed above, what qualities do you think a good researcher must have?

Other qualities of a good researcher

You may have thought of the following:

- **Knowledge** – of the subject that you are researching, of how to undertake research and of yourself, including your strengths and weaknesses.
- **Understanding** – of exactly what it is that you wish to enquire into, of how to undertake research and of yourself, including your strengths and weaknesses. Note that knowledge and understanding are not the same thing – you can know something without really understanding it, but you cannot understand something without knowing it.
- **The ability to work on your own initiative** – this is particularly important if you are undertaking a research study on your own because of the long periods you will be working on your own, collecting or analysing data, but it is also important if you are undertaking research as part of a group.
- **Empathy** – this is particularly important when you are undertaking research into human subjects.
- **Communication skills** – research, even quantitative research, requires the ability to communicate well. This covers not just oral communication, but communication in writing and by numbers. Communication is very important at all stages of the research study, not just whilst doing the research, but at the beginning of the research study when you are trying to 'sell' your ideas to potential sponsors as well as the research and development committee and the research ethics committee, because without their approval you will not be able to go ahead. Similarly, communication is very important at the end of the research because if you cannot communicate your findings simply and effectively to the people to whom it is addressed, whether that be other healthcare professionals, patients or the general public, then your research has little value.
- **A logical and structured mind** – you have to be able to delineate logically the steps that you will be taking in your research study and structure it in such a way that you can be certain that you have covered every aspect and not gone off at a tangent and studied something that bears no relationship to your initial proposal, or have omitted some important steps, thereby making your study virtually worthless.
- **Imagination** – some people think that logic/structure and imagination are incompatible, but a good researcher needs both these skills/attributes. Imagination is essential if you are to make sense of the data you have collected, to be able to make connections between disparate data and see where the data have given rise to other avenues to explore, either during your present study or later.

- **Time** – the ability to make time for, and give time to, your study is crucial to its success. All research takes time, not just in planning, carrying out the research and communicating the findings, but also to stand back from your research and think about it. The good researcher is not just a 'doer' but also a 'thinker'. Taking time out of your busy schedule to step back and think about what you are doing, and to use your imagination as to where your research is taking you, is a very important aspect of undertaking research.

There are others that you can think of if you put your mind to it.

All this may seem quite problematic and you may be wondering how anybody ever becomes a researcher. Well, if you think about the skills that you have as a healthcare professional, you will realise that you already fit the role. All the above skills and attributes are important for healthcare workers, and the only differences between you and a researcher is that a researcher will apply all these skills and attributes to a piece of research, and will have been taught how to do this.

Now, having determined what attributes and skills a researcher needs (and remember, you probably have these to some degree already), in the next section we shall look at the people and organisations involved in research.

Who's who in the world of healthcare research?

'Everyone involved in research with human participants, their organs, tissue or data is responsible for knowing and following the law and the principles of good practice relating to ethics, science, information, health and safety, and finance set out in this framework' (Department of Health 2005: 19. Reproduced under the terms of the Click-Use Licence).

This quotation is from the UK Department of Health's *Research governance framework for health and social work* and sets out the basic responsibility of the people who are concerned with research with humans – which covers all those working in the healthcare professions.

As the document setting out the research governance framework points out, there are many individuals and organisations involved in health or social care research, so this section will briefly discuss these so that you have an idea of the complexity, but more importantly some idea of who can help you, and what their responsibilities are. The Research and Development (R&D) directorate of the DH (2005) has produced a list of the key responsibilities of organisations and individuals involved in research with humans:

- **Researcher** – someone who conducts a research study (you!).
- **Principal/Chief investigator** – this is the person who, when the research is being conducted at one site (e.g. one hospital) by a team of two or more researchers, takes responsibility for the design, conduct and reporting of that research study. However, if the research takes place at more than one site (a multi-site study) and involves two or more researchers, then the chief investigator is the one who takes primary responsibility for the design, conduct and reporting of the research study (whether he/she is an investigator at any particular site).
- **Investigator** – will take responsibility for the conduct of the research study either as an individual (for a one-person study) or as a leader of researchers at one particular site. *Research government framework for health and social care* (2005) makes the very important point that where the study is in the form of a clinical trial involving medicines, then an investigator must be an authorised health professional.

Another point to take note of is that if you are undertaking a research study involving humans as part of an academic qualification, then your academic supervisor is usually classed as your principal or chief investigator.

Key responsibilities of investigators and researchers

1. Developing proposals that are sound, both scientifically and ethically.
2. The submission of the design of, and proposal for, the research study.
3. The submission of the proposed research study for review by an independent research ethics committee.
4. Conducting the research study to the agreed proposal (agreed by Research Governance, Research Ethics and others deemed to have a responsibility for the study) in accordance with legal and ethical requirements and accepted standards of good practice.
5. Providing information for the participants in the study before the research study has begun, so that the participants can make an informed choice as to whether they wish to take part in it.
6. Ensuring the participants' welfare is never compromised.
7. Arranging, at the end of the research, to disseminate the findings and data from the study to interested people.

8. Feeding back the results of the research to the participants (Department of Health 2005: 21–24).

Sponsor

The sponsor is an individual (or an organisation/group) that takes on the responsibility for ensuring that the arrangements for the initiation, management and financing of a research study are in place.

Key responsibilities of sponsors

1. First, the sponsor has to ensure and confirm that everything is ready and in place for the research to commence. This includes:
   - Taking on the responsibility for organising and maintaining the arrangements for the management and funding of the research study.
   - Ensuring that the research protocol, researcher/research team and the research environment are all of a satisfactory scientific and academic quality.
   - Ensuring that ethical approval has been obtained before the research project begins.
   - The final part of this responsibility is only pertinent for clinical trials involving medicines, but in these cases, the sponsor is responsible for seeking the authorisation for the clinical trial and also for making arrangements to investigate 'medicinal products'.
2. The sponsor has to be satisfied that arrangements remain in place throughout the research for ensuring good practice in conducting the study, as well as for the prompt reporting of suspected and/or unexpected adverse events or reactions (Department of Health 2005: 21–24)

Funder

The funder is the organisation or group that provides the funding for a research study.

Key responsibilities of funders

1. The funder is responsible for assessing the quality of the research study as set out in the research proposal.
2. The funder is also responsible for establishing the 'value for money' of the research as detailed in the research proposal.
3. A third responsibility of the funder is to consider the suitability of the research environment, as well as the experience and expertise of the key researchers involved in the research study.

4. Finally, the funder is responsible for requiring that a sponsor takes on the above responsibilities before the research commences (Department of Health 2005: 21–24).

Organisation providing care

This is the organisation responsible for providing health or social care to patients, service users and carers who will be participating in the research study. Before, during and after the research study, all health and social care organisations remain responsible for the quality of care, as well as for the duty of care to anyone taking part in the study and who may be at risk from, or harmed by, any aspect of the research.

Responsible care professional

In a research study, the responsible care professional is any doctor, nurse, social worker, paramedic or other practitioner who is formally responsible for the care of any or all participants whilst they are taking part in the study.

R&D department

This is the department in an organisation that monitors any research taking place within the environment or remit of the organisation.

Research governance committee

This is the committee in an organisation that takes responsibility for the viability of the proposed research study as well as assessing the impact of the research on all people who come within the remit of the organisation, whether patient, professional, client, employee or member of the public. The research cannot commence until this committee has given their permission for it to proceed.

Key responsibilities of the employing organisation
The employing organisation is responsible for:

1. Promoting a culture of quality care within its purview.
2. Ensuring that all the researchers understand their responsibilities and that they discharge these responsibilities with due diligence and professionalism.
3. Ensuring that all research studies are properly designed and that they are submitted for independent review.

4. Ensuring that all studies in their responsibility are managed, monitored and reported on in accordance with the research proposal and protocol.
5. Providing written procedures, training and supervision of all researchers in their employ.
6. Taking action against any suspected misconduct or fraud on the part of the researchers which is brought to their notice (Department of Health 2005: 21–24).

Employing organisation

The employing organisation is the employer of the chief investigator or other researchers. It remains liable for the work of all its employees, including those undertaking research. If an employing organisation holds a contract with a funder for a research study, then that organisation remains responsible for the management of the funds that have been provided by the funder for the research study (Department of Health 2005: 21–24).

Research ethics committee

The research ethics committee is an independent body that provides the participants in a research study, the researchers, the funders, the sponsors, the employers, the organisations providing care and the health and social care professionals with an independent review of whether or not the research proposal that is submitted to it attains recognised ethical standards. No health or social care research study involving humans can take place without the permission of a research ethics committee because the 'dignity, rights, safety and well-being of participants must be the primary consideration in any research study' (Department of Health 2005: 7). Therefore, the Department of Health makes it mandatory that any research that involves humans (patients/clients, service users, care professionals or volunteers), or human organs, tissues or data, has to be reviewed by a research ethics committee in order to ensure that the research meets the required ethical standards (Department of Health 2005: 21–24).

More information and discussion on the very important topic of research ethics will be found in chapter 6.

Participant

A participant is anyone who consents to take part in a research study, whether as a patient, service user, carer, relative of someone who is dead, professional carer, other employee or member of the public. One thing to note is that in legal terms, participants in clinical trials that involve medicines of any description are known as 'subjects' (Department of Health 2005: 21–24).

That concludes the brief look at the people and organisations involved in research. The next section turns to the importance of research in healthcare.

The importance of research to healthcare

To Do

Before reading this section, spend a few minutes thinking about research you have looked at in your field/specialty, and answer these questions:

- What research have you come across?
- Who conducted the research?
- Who was the research aimed at?
- Has the research been implemented in your field or specialty?
- Has the research made a difference to the care you give?
- Do you think that the research has made an important contribution to the care that you give, or that you have seen given by others?
- How did you come to this conclusion?

'Our society is continuously changing. For health, these changes have led to remarkable improvements in the way we identify, diagnose and manage disease. We are now able to consider the prospect of disease prevention through a clear understanding of genetic, social and environmental risk factors and disease processes' (Research and Development Directorate 2005: 4).

As you will discover in chapter 3, all research must have a rationale – a reason for undertaking that particular research study – and there are many 'drivers' that can lead you to consider undertaking a piece of research (a driver is something that 'drives' you to consider and undertake a piece of research). The importance of a piece of research is often linked to the rationale and drivers of the research because if they are linked to such concepts as 'need', 'improvement of care' or 'relief of suffering' rather than 'vanity', 'part of the job', then there is obviously going to be a sound rationale for doing the research.

Those of us who became involved in healthcare many years ago will remember that research was considered as only suitable for doctors and medically qualified academics. Certainly, nurses and other non-doctors were not encouraged to undertake any research – a situation that now seems both archaic and ridiculous. Nowadays it is accepted that everyone who has a stake in the well-being of patients and clients not only can undertake research, but also must actively become involved in research, either as a researcher or as a practitioner who bases their care on the latest evidence and research. We may not wish to carry out our own research, but we should all be capable of, and be prepared to, keep up to date with the latest research related to our jobs and specialties in order to enhance the well-being and care of our patients and clients. Indeed, many healthcare and social care organisa-tions actively encourage everyone in their organisation to take an interest in research as can be seen by the development of research governance/R&D departments in health and social care organisations.

Incidentally, if you wish to find out more about the research that is taking place in your organisation, or are interested in undertaking your own research, a good place to begin is your local R&D/research gov-ernance department. They will be willing to meet you and help you.

The importance of research in health and social care is recognised by the UK government, which has promoted the development of research in these areas for some years now. As Jane Kennedy, Minister for State for Quality and Patient Safety, states in the foreword to the policy consultation document *Best research for best health: A new national health service research strategy – the NHS contribution to health research in England: a consultation*:

> 'Society has high expectations of health and healthcare. Our ability to develop the medicines, care options, and advice on lifestyle choices for the 21st century depends on rigorous applied research. Research also provides us with the evidence to make informed decisions about the benefits and costs of existing health care interventions. It is for these reasons that the Department of Health is a major contributor to health research in the UK with a current annual spend of £650 million' (2005: 4).

Subsequently, Patricia Hewitt (then Secretary of State for Health), wrote: 'Health research provides us with the means to tackle the increasing challenges that disease and ill health are placing on our society' (Research and Development Directorate 2006: 1), and stressed the importance of healthcare research by stating that 'The Government is determined to make the UK the best place in the world for health research, development and innovation' (Research and Development Directorate 2006: 1).

Best research for best health also stresses the importance of research to improving health:

> 'Our focus will be on supporting and funding health-related research, which leads to improved outcomes for people. Evidence from research spanning prevention of ill health, promotion of health, disease management, patient care, delivery of healthcare and its organisation, as well as in public health and social care is key to improving health' (Research and Development Directorate 2006: 4).

Pretty unequivocal!

The government also stresses the importance of inclusion in research (in case you were thinking that all this is only really of importance to doctors) by making the point that,

> 'we seek to include all professionals who have a role in conducting and enabling health research in England, as both leaders and collaborators. We aim to engage patients increasingly in the identification, design, recruitment to, and dissemination of, research projects' (Research and Development Directorate 2006: 4).

After you have read this book and worked through the web program, we hope you will be one of those to answer the government's call.

How to use this book and the accompanying web program

The book and the web program are best used together in order to give you an overall picture of how to prepare a research proposal.

The book

The book is partly concerned with the theory of research and partly with giving you practical tips on how to conduct research. The theory is very important because that gives you the tools to conduct research and also an understanding of research. You have read above that anyone can be a researcher because everyone has the innate ability to be a researcher. Unfortunately, though, to be a good researcher you need something to complement and develop this innate ability, and this is what a knowledge and understanding of the theory of research can do for you. Consequently, the chapters are arranged in the same order in which you will develop your research proposal because, as the title of this book and web program stress, our aim is to help you to produce a research proposal.

A research proposal is probably the most important aspect of research that researchers consider and produce in order to undertake a satisfactory piece of research. Unfortunately, experience has shown that many potential researchers are put off undertaking research because they find producing a research proposal that is acceptable to the various people and organisations (as discussed above) needed to sanction your potential research is so testing. That is why we have produced this book and web program in order to help and encourage you to produce a research proposal that will successfully pass through all the stages before you can start your actual research.

With this in mind, the chapters are not only arranged in the same order in which you would develop and write a research proposal, they are also linked closely to the web program, so that if you work through both the book and the web program you could have your own research proposal ready to submit to the various organisations and committees (as detailed above).

The chapters

The chapters commence with a theoretical discussion before looking at more practical issues of how to undertake research, and in order are:

- **Chapter 1: Research and allied concepts** – this chapter examines and discusses what research is and how it differs from similar practices and concepts, particularly clinical audit, clinical effectiveness and evidence-based practice. Many people in health and social care confuse these concepts and practices.
- **Chapter 2: Philosophical assumptions** – introduces you to the philosophical assumptions underlying the research process. Whilst this is a very theoretical chapter, understanding it will allow you to make sense of the practical aspects of undertaking research.
- **Chapter 3: Developing the question** – before you get as far as writing and developing your research study, it is very important that you are clear about what exactly it is that you wish to research. Therefore, it is very important, if not absolutely essential, that you develop a good, clear research question, because once you have that fixed it is much easier to start to develop your proposal and your actual research, because you have an accurate and unambiguous idea of what you wish to study. This chapter discusses ways in which you can develop your research question.
- **Chapter 4: Reviewing the literature** – once you have determined your research question, the next stage in preparing for and writing your research proposal is to review the literature about your proposed topic of interest. This is partly so that you know what has been written (to avoid your covering old ground) and partly to give

you ideas of what needs to be looked at and how you can do this. Again, this chapter gives you practical information and techniques on how to find and review literature.

- **Chapter 5: Research design** – if you have worked out your research question, it should be quite easy to determine how you will design your research study. This chapter gives you information on the different types of research methodologies and designs, so that you can select the most appropriate to answer your research question.

- **Chapter 6: Ethics** – a major hurdle for all potential researchers is getting their research proposal through a research ethics committee. This is because, as mentioned above, all research involving humans (or parts of humans) has to be submitted to, and receive approval from, an independent research committee. This can be very difficult, depending on the topic of your research and the methodology. This chapter examines what we mean by ethics and, linked to the web program, gives practical advice on how to discuss the ethics of your research in your research proposal.

- **Chapter 7: Selecting participants** – this depends on your research question and design. In this chapter, the various methods of selecting participants for your proposed research are discussed.

- **Chapter 8: Collecting data** – in this chapter you will find information on how to collect data for your proposed research. Different types of data collection methods are discussed, so that you will be able to choose the most appropriate one for your research and that will answer your research question.

- **Chapter 9: Analysing data** – having collected your data, the next stage is to analyse the information. This chapter explains how you can go about this, using practical examples.

- **Chapter 10: Communicating research findings** – having completed your research project, you will want to communicate your findings to all who may be interested in them. This chapter explains how you can do this and offers practical advice on presenting at conferences and writing for publication.

- **Chapter 11: Current research issues in healthcare** – to complete the book, the final chapter discusses various current research issues that are much discussed within the subject of healthcare, including:
  - the ethics of undertaking research using human subjects, embryos and animal subjects;
  - the availability, origins and provenance of funding;
  - the problem of vested interests and their potential implications regarding the funding, the process, and the reporting of research;
  - the politicisation of research;
  - the implementation of research findings.

All of these points have to be considered, discussed and defended when you write your research proposal, so it is important that you have knowledge and understanding about them if your proposed research is ever to be realised.

Finally, there are activities and scenarios for you to work through, which will increase your understanding of research and research proposals.

The web program

The first thing to say about the web program is that it is integral to the book – they go together and are best studied together. The web program supplements the book chapters to give you an opportunity to work through the experience of preparing an actual or virtual research proposal.

Aims of the web program

The aims of this web program are:

- to introduce you to the writing of research proposals;
- to enable you to write a research proposal of your own.

How to navigate through the web program

The web program works through all the aspects of producing a research proposal and is very easy to navigate, even if you do not consider yourself computer-literate. Everything works by just one click of a mouse, and to navigate through the various sections, you just need to click on the contents that are to be found in the column on the side of every one of the web pages and headed 'CONTENTS', as shown in the box.

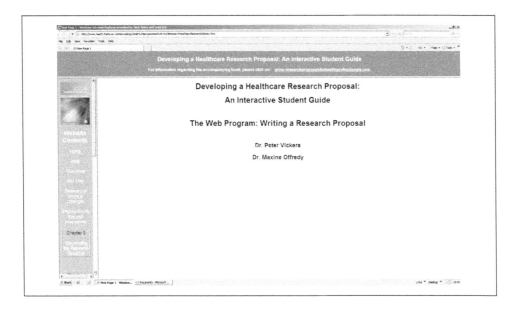

These are just a few of the contents of the web program. When you click on one of these content hyperlinks (e.g. Title), you will either be taken to a page like the one below (the script is much larger and easier to read in the actual web program) or to a page similar to the one in the second box below (depending on the actual content of the section).

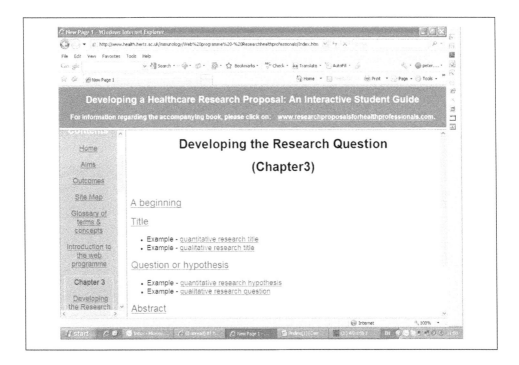

From this, by clicking on to a hyperlink you will be taken to a page similar to the one below or the actual contents hyperlink will take you straight to a page similar to the one below:

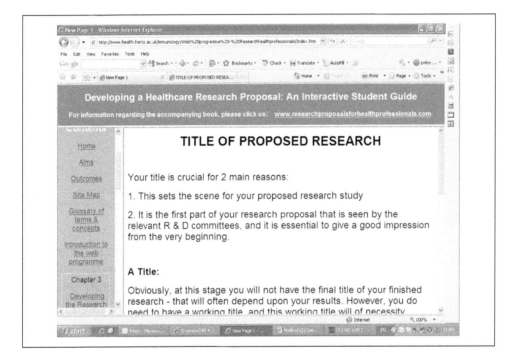

Within the web pages there are hyperlinks that you can click on. You will recognise a hyperlink because:

- It is in blue – a different colour from the rest of the text.
- It is underlined.
- When you place your pointer over the hyperlink word, it changes from an arrow into a hand.

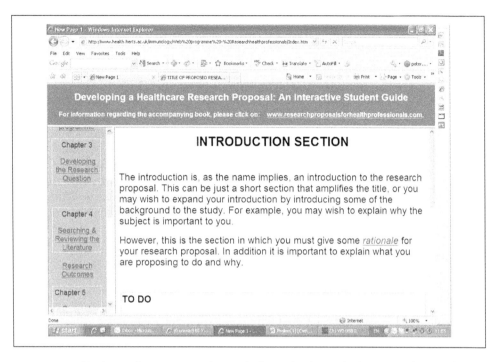

In the web program, if you click on the hyperlink 'rationale' (as shown above), you will be taken to a web page (as shown below) that discusses what we mean by the term and its importance in a research proposal, as well as some idea of how you can structure your section on the rationale for your proposed research.

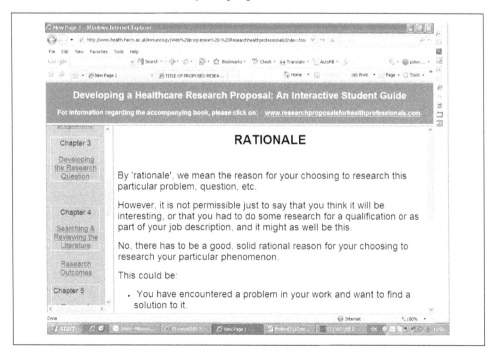

You can return to the previous page by clicking on the appropriate hyperlink on the web page (in the example above, if you click on 'introduction section', you will return to that page), by clicking on the return arrow at the top of your computer screen or by clicking on the appropriate hyperlink in the 'contents' column.

In addition to the information given in the web program, at each stage you will be presented with the appropriate section of two successful research proposals – one for a qualitative research study and one for a quantitative research study – so that you will constantly have these by you to help you to structure your own proposal.

That is all there is to navigating and working through the web program. If you work through the web program in conjunction with this book, you can easily finish up with your own research proposal.

Summary

This introduction and the web program have set the scene for you as you start to learn about research and how to write a research proposal.

All, that remains is to tell you to enjoy the experience. There is great satisfaction to be had in undertaking research and, as we have stressed, we all have the ability to undertake good research that will help to improve the care we give to our patients and clients – which is what we all wish to do. This book and the web program will give you the tools you need to improve the care that you give your patients and clients.

Good luck, and have fun with your research!

References

Department of Health (2005) *Research governance framework for health and social care* (2nd edition). London, DH. http://www.dh.gov.uk/en/ Publicationsandstatistics/Publications/PublicationsPolicyAndGuidance/ DH_4108962.

Research and Development Directorate (2005) *Best research for best health: A new national health service research strategy – the NHS contribution to health research in England: a consultation.* London: DH. http://www.dh.gov.uk/ en/Consultations/Closedconsultations/DH_4121788.

Research and Development Directorate (2006) *Best research for best health: A new national health research strategy* London: DH. http://www.dh.gov.uk/en/ Publicationsandstatistics/Publications/PublicationsPolicyAndGuidance/ DH_4127127.

Research and Allied Concepts

Introduction

This book is designed to develop your appreciation of some of the key features of research methodologies and approaches. By completing the exercises in this book, you will gain a better knowledge and understanding of the research processes involved. From the outset we should state that this book is for healthcare professionals and students who are new to research and, therefore, we have assumed that you have no prior knowledge of research. Consequently, we have avoided using unnecessary jargon that may confuse you and make it difficult for you to feel confident about undertaking your own research proposal. After all, that is the most interesting and important part of your involvement with 'research'.

To begin with, this chapter offers some definitions and discussions about:

* research;
* clinical audit;
* comparison of clinical audit and research;
* clinical effectiveness; and
* evidence-based practice.

The discussions in this chapter are put into context and discussed within the current healthcare climate. The chapter concludes with activities relating to practice for you to undertake. These, and the activities in the other chapters, will help you to understand fully the content of the chapters by your undertaking something related to them.

What is research?

Let us start at the very beginning and discuss what we mean by 'research'.

The word 'research' is frequently used in everyday conversations, but has different meanings according to the context in which it is used. This chapter specifically relates to research undertaken within a healthcare context. In healthcare we are always looking for answers to questions that are related to the health and well-being of our patients/clients. For example, we may wish to find answers to questions such as:

* What are patients' perspectives concerning a new type of treatment?
* How does the effectiveness of one type of wound dressing compare with that of another?
* How do healthcare professionals feel about working in a multi-disciplinary team?

And so on.

So, from what you have just read, you can see that research begins with a question. Now, you may think that we know the answers to some of these questions – and you may be right – but unless we subject these answers to a scientific process, then our knowledge and understanding could be said to be intuitive at best, and at worst quite possibly be based on guesswork and hunches.

The role of research, therefore, is to provide a systematic framework for obtaining answers to questions by studying and gathering the evidence in a scientific manner. In other words, the process of arriving at an answer to a question in the context of healthcare research has to follow certain rules. These rules are set out in different philosophies which underpin the type of research that is being undertaken. By following these rules our research can be judged by others to be objective, valid and reliable – three important tests of how good a piece of research is. So, to simplify: research is a way of thinking about a problem in a systematic and scientific way. We call this way of thinking about a problem a **research process**.

We can now take a few moments to look at the stages of the research process (see Table 1.1). As you can see from Table 1.1, the process of undertaking research involves eight stages which we need to work through when preparing a research proposal and doing the research study itself. These eight stages are:

1. Conceptual – conceiving your proposed study (chapters 1 and 2).
2. Question/hypothesis formulation – how you set about determining the question or hypothesis that will need to be answered or proved/disproved by the research (chapter 3).

3. The formulation of aims and objectives – these are very important because they follow the determining of the research question or hypothesis, and they let you set out what you hope to achieve with your research study within the context of the research question or hypothesis (chapter 3).
4. The planning and design of the research study – this is where you ask (and answer) the questions: Why are we doing this research? How are we going to do it? Where are we going to do it? You will need to make a number of decisions about how you are going to set about answering your research question or proving/disproving your hypothesis (chapter 5).
5. Collecting data – this stage consists of your collecting the data for your research study in order to achieve your aims and objectives as well as answer your research question or prove/disprove your hypothesis (chapter 8).
6. Analysing your data – this is the part of the study where you start to make sense of the data you have collected. Analysing your data will allow you to answer your research question or prove/disprove your hypothesis. However, this is not the end of your research; the next stage, presenting your research findings, is an important part of any research study (chapter 9).
7. Presenting your results and findings – this is the stage in which you organise your findings in such a way that they are clear, interesting, accessible, understandable and relevant to others who may read the report of your research study (chapter 10).
8. Disseminating your results – this is the final stage of your research when you send your results to all relevant and interested people/organisations, by writing papers and/or presenting them at conferences (chapter 10).

You may have come across some words that are new to you in this list, but do not worry, as you work through this book and the accompanying web program, you will become familiar with all these terms, and many others, and understand them and their significance to the process of undertaking and reading research studies. If you think of research as being a foreign language, then, just as you have to learn a new vocabulary and grammar, and their contexts, so it is with learning about research. Research has its own vocabulary and 'grammar' (methodology and philosophy) and you have to learn these within the context of a research study. Similarly, just as it is better and much easier to learn a foreign language when you are living with it – for example, living in the country where the language you are studying is spoken – so you will learn about research and understand it much better and far more easily if you are learning it in a 'live' situation – when doing some research. This is the reason for encouraging and helping you to write a research proposal (whether for an actual research

Table 1.1 Stages of research.

Stage 1	What?	
Conceptual		This involves thinking, reading, theorising, rethinking and discussing your ideas with colleagues and experts in the field or in your area of interest.
Stage 2 Question/ hypothesis formulation		At this point, you would be reading the related literature to (i) get an idea of what has been done and how it has been done; (ii) assess the results of the research and gaps in the literature; and (iii) formulate your question/hypothesis which will provide direction for the research. (A hypothesis is a tentative statement to explain observations or facts and which requires experimental investigation for verification.)
Stage 3 Formulate aims and objectives		Aims are statements of what the research sets out to achieve. In other words, what do you want to find out?
		Objectives are a set of specific statements pertaining to the aim of the research and must fulfil the requirements of the aim. Aims and objectives are therefore interrelated and the latter can be seen as being more detailed information about the aims. They are the intellectual activities that the researcher will perform throughout the research process.
Stage 4 Design and planning	**How? Whom? Where?**	The researcher must make a number of decisions about how to go about doing the research. These methodological decisions have implications for the *validity* and *credibility* of the study findings. If the methods used to collect and analyse the data are flawed, then the conclusions will be flawed also and doubtful. At this stage of the research process, you will be involved in:

- *Selecting the research design*: i.e. the overall plan, how to get answers to the question being studied and how to handle some of the difficulties encountered in the study.
- *Thinking about a theoretical framework*: you may wish to use a theoretical framework to structure and analyse the research.
- *Identifying the population* to be studied.
- *Selecting measures for the research variables*: i.e. defining the research variables and clarifying exactly what each means.
- *Designing the sampling plan*: decide on your sample and how you will collect data, bearing in mind time and cost, and level of skill required. Sampling procedures include probability sampling and non-probability sampling (these are discussed later in the book).
- *Deciding on location.*
- *Finalising and reviewing the research plan*: showing your research plan to colleagues to get constructive criticism. The research plan is sometimes referred to as the research proposal.
- *Ethical considerations*: you will need to discuss this with your R&D lead (or their equivalent) to ascertain what other approval may be required. Approval **must** be obtained **before** data collection.
- *Pilot study*, if appropriate.

Table 1.1 (*Continued*)

Stage 5 Empirical stage – data collection	How?	This involves the collection of the data and approaches used to answer the research question/hypothesis. More than one method may be used; the commonest are interviews and questionnaires.
Stage 6 Analytic stage	How?	This is the process of systematically explaining the data so that their meaning, structure and relationships are clearly articulated. The analysis will depend on whether the approach used is quantitative or qualitative. The key point is that the information gathered will be transformed so that it provides useful information and lets you reach conclusions. Qualitative data involve integration and synthesis of narrative data, whereas quantitative data are analysed through statistical procedures to describe, summarise and compare data. Whatever approach you use, the analysis must be carried out in relation to the research problem.
Stage 7 Presentation of results/findings	How?	You should put a lot of thought into how you present your results or findings. For example, consider whether figures or graphs are the best way to bring out your data and whether these will help the reader follow what you have found. Tables are also useful for presenting information as they can provide a complete picture for the reader.
Stage 8 Dissemination	How?	Results of data are of little use if they are not communicated to others. Ideally, the final step of a first-class study is to plan for its utilisation in practice.

study or as a virtual project) as you work through the accompanying web program.

The other thing to point out about the list on pages 2–4 and Table 1.1 is that all these stages are covered fully in this book by being assigned a whole chapter so that we can introduce you to the eight stages and help you to understand them as you work though the book and accompanying web program.

At this stage, it is important to stress that the research proposal is essential to the whole process of undertaking research because it encapsulates everything that we need to go through in order to undertake a research study. Consequently, the better the proposal, the better and easier is the process of undertaking a research study. It is this process of absorbing information, knowledge and understanding in its natural and 'live' context that is the rationale for this book and web program, both of which are focused on helping you to prepare a research proposal.

The next section discusses the 'audit' and explains the differences between research and audit.

What is clinical audit?

Many healthcare students undertaking a project as part of their degree programme, or other academic studies – and indeed many qualified healthcare professionals who wish to look at a problem in their own practice – are uncertain if their work will be classified as research or as an audit, as the two activities are closely related. For example, they both:

- involve questions relating to quality of care;
- can be done prospectively (looking forward) or retrospectively (looking back);
- use:
  - sampling,
  - questionnaires,
  - the analysis of findings;
- are usually professionally led.

Nevertheless, audit and research are very different processes.

The National Institute for Health and Clinical Excellence (2002: 1) defines an audit as a:

'quality improvement process that seeks to improve patient care and outcomes through systematic review of care against explicit criteria and the implementation of change. Aspects of the structures, processes and outcomes of care are selected and systematically evaluated against explicit criteria. Where indicated, changes are implemented at an individual, team or service level and further monitoring is used to confirm improvement in healthcare delivery.'

An earlier UK government White Paper, *Working for Patients* (Secretary of State for Health (1989: 39), describes medical audit as:

'a systematic, critical analysis of the quality of medical care, including the procedures used for diagnosis and treatment, the use of resources, and the resulting outcome for the patient.'

The Healthcare Commission (2004) expands this:

> 'The overall aim of clinical audit is to improve patient outcomes by improving professional practice and the general quality of services delivered. This is achieved through a continuous process where healthcare professionals review patient care against agreed standards and make changes, where necessary, to meet those standards. The audit is then repeated to see if the changes have been made and the quality of patient care improved' (http://www.healthcarecommission.org.uk/ihealthcareproviders/serviceprovidersinformation/nationalclinicalaudit.cfn).

Whereas,

> 'Research is the attempt to derive generalisable knowledge by addressing clearly defined questions with systematic and rigorous methods' (Department of Health 2005: 3).

In other words, research is the systematic process of collecting and analysing information to increase our understanding of the topic being investigated. The researcher is therefore charged with contributing to knowledge. (If you are uncertain or concerned at this stage, then go back to the earlier discussion in this chapter about research.)

The method or process that we use in clinical audit is called the clinical audit cycle, whereas in research it is the research process, as outlined in Table 1.1 above.

The clinical audit cycle is a process of continuous improvement within the context of healthcare and treatment. The purpose of the clinical audit cycle is to identify problems and ask questions about healthcare practice in order to help healthcare practitioners reflect, review and act so that they can start to resolve these problems and questions, and so make changes that will improve patient/client care. It is called a clinical audit because it is often represented as an audit cycle or spiral, in which, following the identification of a problem or asking a question, the following processes are put into practice:

1. Setting and putting into practice a standard related to the problem/question, which it is hoped will improve the care/treatment offered by healthcare practitioners in a specialty/environment.
2. Determining and putting into practice action to meet the standard to improve the care/treatment.
3. The development of an audit tool to help to determine whether the standard that is now in practice is being met.
4. The collection of data concerned with the problem/question using the audit tool that has been developed to determine whether or not there has been any improvement in care/treatment as a result of the standard being implemented.
5. The analysis and interpretation of the data collected in stage 3 above.

6. Confirmation of the standard and the action to achieve that standard, if it has been met.

Thus the circle has been closed: initial poor practice → action/standard to improve the practice → audit of the standard/action → confirmation of the standard/action → carry on with the improved care/treatment.

However, if the action has not improved the care/treatment and so has not achieved the standard, then the clinical audit cycle becomes a clinical audit spiral, because the circle is not closed. Instead, the audit process continues in this way:

7. Determining what action to take if the standard has not been met and the care has not improved.
8. Putting into place new/amended action to improve the situation.
9. Re-auditing, analysing and interpreting the data that have been collected from the second audit.
10. Either confirming the new action because it has met the standard or repeating the whole process by changing the action, and so on.
11. Doing this until the standard has been met or looking at the standard again – it may not be achievable in that situation and so may need modifying, in which case you then repeat the modified/new clinical audit cycle/spiral until it has been met.

Basically, clinical audit is used to compare current practice with evidence of good practice, and so it is used to make changes that improve the delivery of care.

To Do

This brief look at clinical audit may seem complicated at first so, using the principle that we learn and understand better by 'doing' rather than 'seeing' or 'reading', use the information above to draw your own clinical audit cycle/spiral about some aspect of care in your practice, which should encompass all the points discussed.

After all that, we can now turn our attention to the main differences between clinical audit and research. These are outlined in Table 1.2, which summarises the differences.

However, research and audit, whilst being discrete processes (i.e. they can operate independently, without the other), also have common links and can work together to improve the care we offer to our patients/clients.

Table 1.2 Differences between research and clinical audit.

Research	Clinical audit
Creates new knowledge about what works and what does not	Answers the question, 'Are we following best practice?'
Is based on a hypothesis	Measures against standards
Is **usually** carried out on a large scale over a long period	Is **usually** carried out on a relatively small population over a short time span
May involve patients receiving completely new treatment	**Never** involves a completely new treatment
May involve experiments on patients	**Never** involves anything being done to patients beyond their normal clinical management
May involve patients being allocated to different treatment groups	**Never** involves allocation of patients to different treatment groups
Is based on a scientifically valid sample size (this may not apply to pilot studies)	Depending on circumstances, **may** be pragmatically based on a sample size that is acceptable to senior clinicians
Always requires ethics approval	Does not require ethics approval
Results are generalisable and hence publishable	Results are relevant within the local setting only (although the audit process may be of interest to a wider audience; hence audits are also published)
Findings influence the activities of clinical practice as a whole	Findings influence activities of local clinicians and teams

Reproduced from *British Medical Journal* (1992), 305, pp. 905–6 with permission from BMJ Publishing Group.

We can summarise the link between audit and research like this:

- Clinical audit can be seen as the final stage of a research study, that is, the study is implemented and then audited for its effectiveness.
- Undertaking an audit can highlight areas for research, and vice versa.
- Undertaking an audit can highlight whether research evidence is lacking.
- The audit process is part of the dissemination of evidence-based practice.

So much for the links between audit and research. There are also differences, which are summed up by the United Bristol Healthcare Trust (2008) in three questions for potential researchers/auditors:

1. Are you undertaking this project because you want to improve the quality of patient care in your local setting?
2. Will your project compare current practice with established standards?
3. Will your project involve changes to treatment or services?

The Trust suggests that if your answer is 'yes' to the first two questions and 'no' to the third, then it is likely that the project is a clinical audit. If your response is different from what has been suggested, your project may be research, in which case you will need ethics approval (http://hospital.blood.co.uk/library/pdf/safe_use/The_Difference_between_Clinical_Audit_and_Research.pdf (see chapter 6 and the web program).

Is that clear? Can you see how the two processes – clinical audit and research – differ, but at the same time can be complementary?

Reflection

Think of an audit that you have carried out, or one that has been been carried out by others in your practice (ward, unit or other place of work). Now reflect on the following questions:

- What was the audit about?
- Who organised and undertook it?
- How did they do it?
- What was the result? Was the practice satisfactory or were there problems in the care/treatment that the audit highlighted?
- What happened next?

Next, we turn to another process that is linked to research and audit: service evaluation. You may already have encountered this; if not, you probably will encounter it at a future stage in your practice.

Service evaluation

A question students, as well as qualified healthcare professionals, often ask is whether service evaluation is the same as clinical audit. Harris & Hardman (2001: 70) provide a useful definition:

'A service evaluation is a type of applied research which investigates the effectiveness and appropriateness of a particular service, i.e. is it achieving what it set out to do?'

In other words, undertaking a service evaluation means assessing sys-tematically all the important steps involved in any field of healthcare service. As a consequence, the method(s) used to evaluate a service should provide enough information to let us know whether or not the service should continue. It may employ elements of research and clinical audit, and it consists of one or more of the following:

- qualitative or quantitative data (see chapter 5 and the web program);
- aspects of the research process, for example, the collection of additional data (see chapter 8 and the web program);
- cost-benefit analysis;
- identification of strengths and limitations of the service.

To give you some idea of the processes of research, clinical audit and service evaluation Table 1.3 gives examples of different studies using research, clinical audit and service evaluation: Referring to Table 1.3a, try to work out which of the three processes – clinical audit, service evaluation or research – would be used for each of the three questions or problems, then check the answers in Table 1.3b. If you didn't arrive at the right solution, try to figure out where you went wrong.

Did you get all three right? If not, try to work out where you went wrong, but this time use Table 1.4, which summarises the difference between research, audit and service evaluation.

Table 1.3a   Topics illustrating type of studies.

Topic	Type of study
What is the association between women with breast cancer and smoking?	
To decide whether targets set by the government are being achieved: All patients telephoning a GP surgery are offered an appointment within 48 hours	
Data collection: (a) from service users to see if the service is appropriate for their needs; and (b) from staff about various aspects of the new service.	

Table 1.3b   Topics illustrating type of studies.

Topic	Type of study
What is the association between women with breast cancer and smoking?	Research study
To decide whether targets set by the government are being achieved. All patients telephoning a GP surgery are offered an appointment within 48 hours	Clinical audit
Data collection: (a) from service users to see if the service is appropriate for their needs; and (b) from staff about various aspects of the new service	Service evaluation

Table 1.4 Difference between research, audit and service evaluation.

Research	Clinical audit	Service evaluation
Creates new knowledge about what works and what does not	Answers the question, 'Are we following best practice?'	Undertaken solely to define or assess current care
Is based on a hypothesis	Measures against standards	Measures current service without reference to a standard
Is **usually** carried out on a large scale over a prolonged period	Is **usually** carried out on a relatively small population over a short time span	Size of the evaluation is variable
May involve patients receiving a completely new treatment	**Never** involves a completely new treatment	**Never** involves a completely new treatment
May involve experiments on patients	**Never** involves anything being done to patients beyond their normal clinical management	**Usually** involves analysis of existing data but may include administration of interview or questionnaire
May involve patients being allocated to different treatment groups	**Never** involves allocation of patients to different treatment groups	**Never** involves allocation of patients to different treatment groups
Is based on a scientifically valid sample size (this may not apply to pilot studies)	Depending on circumstances, **may** be pragmatically based on a sample size	Depending on circumstances, **may** be pragmatically based on a sample size
Results are generalisable and hence publishable	Results are relevant within local setting only (although the audit process may be of interest to a wider audience and hence audits are also published)	Results are relevant within a local setting only (although the audit process may be of interest to a wider audience and hence audits are also published)
Findings influence the activities of clinical practice as a whole	Findings influence activities of local clinicians and teams	Findings influence activities of local clinicians and teams

Although any of these may raise ethical issues, under current Guidance (National Research Ethics Service 2007), the following applies for each of them.

Always requires ethics approval	Does not require ethics approval	Does not require ethics approval

Source: Adapted with permission from NHS National Patient Safety Agency /National Research Ethics Service (2007) and Smith (1992).

Scenario

You are working in the community caring for people with drug addictions and HIV. You find that people are not coming to see you at your 'drop-in' centre.

- How would you find out why?
- Which method would you use – research, clinical audit or service evaluation?
- Why?

Possible suggestions can be found at the end of this chapter.

Issues to consider when undertaking research, audit and service evaluation

There are four very important principles to consider that are common to all three processes discussed in this chapter, and these all come under the heading of 'confidentiality'. They are:

1. Confidentiality – patient confidentiality must be ensured at all times.
2. Data Protection Act 1998 – the data collected should be adequate, relevant and not excessive. The data should be stored securely and not kept for longer than necessary.
3. Caldicott Principles – patient-identifiable data must only be collected and/or transferred for justifiable purposes.
4. Good practice in clinical audit suggests that data about a patient should be assigned a unique identification code rather than using the patient's personal details.

You will come across these in different guises throughout this book and the web program, but mainly you will explore them in chapter 6. However, the summary above introduces you to the important concepts of confidentiality and anonymity.

The next sections of this chapter explore two other methods of ensuring that you employ best practice in your work: clinical effectiveness and evidence-based practice. We start with a discussion of evidence-based practice.

Evidence-based practice

Confusion may lie in understanding what evidence-based practice (EBP) is – i.e. what it is and where it sits in relation to research, clinical audit and service evaluation.

Sackett et al.'s (1996: 71) often quoted definition of evidence-based practice can answer these questions. It states that EBP is:

'the conscientious, explicit and judicious use of current best evidence about the care of individual patients. The practice of evidence-based healthcare means integrating individual clinical expertise with the best available external, clinical evidence from systematic research.'

This strategy has been applied to the broader practice of healthcare, including nursing and the allied health practices. The demand for high quality care has come from a number of sources, including government, patients and their carers, the public and the nursing profession. This demand is accompanied by organisational change in healthcare provision and the need to ensure that limited resources are used to provide healthcare that is based on the best available evidence (Department of Health 1998).

So we can see that EBP is not research, but rather is gathering evidence to allow us to provide the best possible care, although it may not have been subject to a formal research study.

Evidence-based practice has five stages:

1. The development of clear questions arising from the patient's problem.
2. These questions are used to search the literature for evidence relating to the problem.
3. This evidence is appraised critically for its validity and usefulness.
4. The best available current evidence, together with clinical expertise and the patient's perspectives, are used to provide care.
5. Patient outcomes are evaluated through the process of audit, peer assessment (including self-evaluation) or the research process.

These stages are explained in chapters 3 and 4.

Clinical effectiveness

Clinical effectiveness is a general term that covers the provision of care in accordance with quality improvement methods such as clinical audit, evidence-based clinical guidelines, benchmarking, standards, practice development and research (Department of Health 2004, National Institute for Clinical Excellence 2002).

Clinical effectiveness has been defined as:

'The extent to which clinical interventions, when deployed in the field for a particular patient or population, do what they are intended to do – i.e. maintain and improve health and secure the greatest possible health gain from the available resources' (NHS Executive 1996).

In other words, clinical effectiveness is about doing the right thing, to the right person, at the right time, and is concerned with demonstrating improvements in quality performance, care/treatment, effectiveness and cost effectiveness – i.e. giving patients total quality experience of their care (Effectiveness Matters 2001).

The steps for improving effectiveness in clinical practice are:

- Producing and accessing the evidence that already exists (e.g. looking at research, patterns of care and population needs). In other words, it is not concerned with providing new evidence as research, for example, does.
- Reviewing and changing practice, for example, then the use of clinical audit, benchmarking and national guidelines.
- Monitoring and evaluation (e.g. measuring health benefits and health improvement, patient and carer experience) (NHS Executive 1996).

Clinical effectiveness comes in five parts. These are included to introduce you to the topic of clinical effectiveness, but as clinical effectiveness is not a part of our aim, which is to introduce you to, and help you to write, research proposals. This is only a brief look at what clinical effectiveness means.

Selecting a specific aspect of practice to explore

1. Obtaining evidence from:
   - research journals;
   - databases;
   - national-level studies based on research, e.g. clinical guidelines (National Institute for Clinical Excellence [NICE]);
   - systematic reviews;
   - national standard frameworks (NSFs); and
   - professional networks.
2. Implementing the evidence by changing practice to include the research evidence and where possible adapting national standards or guidelines to suit local circumstances.
3. Ensuring that you are providing best practice on a day-to-day basis, as well as pointing you in the direction of making improvements in your practice.
4. Evaluating the impact of the changed practice and readjusting practice as necessary, usually through clinical audit and patient feedback.

A number of studies have already been undertaken in the practice settings to assess clinical effectiveness. Here are just two of them to give you a flavour of what is possible.

Harvey (2004) used clinical performance information to underpin quality improvement strategy for her clinical area. Patients and staff

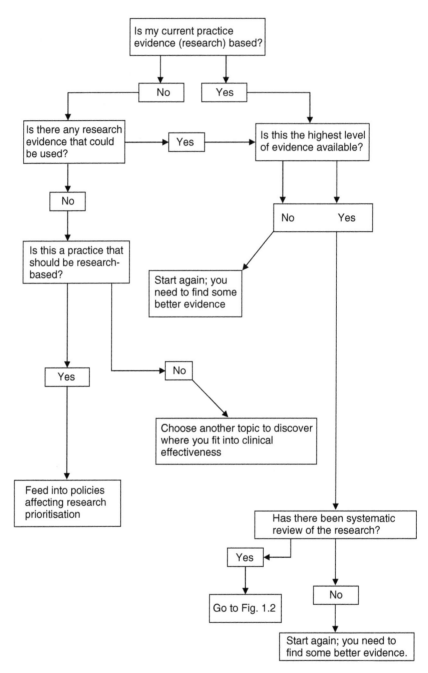

Figure 1.1   Clinical effectiveness – checking your practice is evidence-based (adapted from McClarey & Duff (1997))

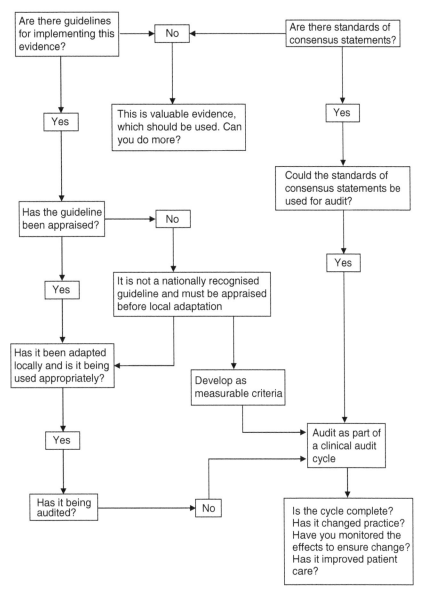

Figure 1.2 Implementing and auditing change (adapted from McClarey & Duff (1997))

were involved in the development of a clinical effectiveness framework and Healthcare and Trust-specific indicators to monitor the quality and effectiveness of healthcare at a system-wide level.

Woods (2006) used a mixed-methods approach to explore the initial management and treatment of neonates by experienced consultant neonatologists and advanced neonatal nurse practitioners. The analysis showed no statistical difference in the standard and quality of care provided by the two categories of healthcare staff in the majority of areas evaluated. However, Woods found that trends in the data suggest that the nurses did not perform as well as the medical consultants in terms of the overall completeness or comprehensiveness of the standard of care provided in a number of areas.

Summary

This chapter has offered discussion and explanations of the following key concepts:

- research;
- clinical audit;
- service evaluation;
- evidence-based practice;
- clinical effectiveness.

In addition, it has demonstrated the differences between research, clinical audit and service evaluation and provided examples of how to distinguish whether a proposal can be classified as research, clinical audit or service evaluation. The activities below are intended to embed the information in this chapter into the reality of the workplace.

Activities

Activity 1

- Explain what you understand by research, clinical audit, service evaluation and evidence-based practice.
- From your own experience, explain the barriers to the use of evidence-based practice, using the following headings:
  - the individual;
  - the organisation;
  - the environment.

Activity 2

Using the checklist provided in Figures 1.1 and 1.2, ascertain whether your practice is evidence-based/clinically effective. Compile a list of some of the causes or barriers to evidence-based/clinically effective practice.

- Why is clinical effectiveness important?
- What impact does it have on your clinical activities?
- How many times have you changed your practice in the last two years?

References and further reading

Department of Health (1993) *Clinical audit – meeting and improving standards in health care*. London: DH.

Department of Health (1998) *A first class service: quality in the new NHS*. London: DH.

Department of Health (2004) *Standards for better health*. London: DH.

Department of Health (2005) *Research governance framework for health and social care* (second edition). London: DH.

Effectiveness Matters (2001) *Accessing the evidence on clinical effectiveness* **5**(1). York: York Centre for Review and Dissemination.

Harris R. & Harman E. (2001) A formative model of service evaluation. *Journal of Clinical Excellence* **3**: 69–73.

Harvey R. (2004) Using clinical performance information to improve the quality of care in a specialist NHS trust. *Journal of Nursing Management* **12**: 427–435.

McClarey M. & Duff L. (1997) Clinical effectiveness and evidence-based practice. *Nursing Standard* **11**: 33–37.

National Institute for Clinical Excellence (2002) *Principles for best practice in clinical audit*. London: Radcliffe Medical Press.

NHS Executive (1996) *Promoting clinical effectiveness: a framework for action in and through the NHS*. Leeds: DH.

NHS National Patient Safety Agency (2007) *National research ethics service*. London: National Patient Safety Agency.

Sackett D. L., Rosenberg W., Gray J. A., Haynes R. B. & Richardson W. S. (1996) Evidence-based medicine: what it is and what it isn't. *British Medical Journal* **312**: 71–72.

Secretary of State for Health (1989) *Working for patients*. Cmnd, 555. London: HMSO.

Smith R. (1992) Audit & research. *British Medical Journal* **305**: 905–906.

Woods L. (2006) Evaluating the clinical effectiveness of neonatal nurse practitioners: an exploratory study. *Journal of Clinical Nursing* **15**(1): 35–44.

Scenario – Possible suggestions/answers

This is a tricky one, and the simple answer is that you could use any of the three processes depending on what you were looking at. For example:

Research: You may decide that you are going to ask people with drug dependency and HIV in the community – in other words, your target group (as well as other community workers) what they think the reason is, and also what would encourage them to attend. This would probably be a qualitative research project, using a phenomenological approach (see chapters 2 and 5 and the web program).

Clinical audit: If you already have a standard, you may wish to develop an audit tool and measure your actual practice against the standard. In this way you may see what you are doing inappropriately and change your practice accordingly. If, on the other hand, there is no standard, then you will need to look at setting a standard for your practice. This could involve contacting others performing a similar role elsewhere in the country and seeing if they have standards you can use; if not, working with a group and setting your own standards which you can then put into practice, and later audit.

Service evaluation: You may decide to do a full service evaluation to see if the service you are providing is of any real merit. Perhaps there is no need of the service in your area, or it is in the wrong place, or the opening hours are not suitable for the potential clientele. You would also look at the cost – is it worthwhile, given the attendance? Could the money be utilised in a different service, whilst still helping the potential clientele? Can you identify the strengths and weaknesses (or limitations) of what you are offering?

So you can see that the method you opt to use – research, clinical audit or service evaluation – depends on what you want to examine in the service that you wish to provide/are providing. This is a useful lesson for you to absorb for when you come to look at the methodology of research and have to decide which type of research you are going to undertake.

Philosophical Assumptions

Introduction

This chapter introduces you to the philosophical assumptions, or set of beliefs, that underlie the research process.

Philosophy

You have come across this word 'philosophy' several times in chapter 1 and you will continue to meet it in the following chapters. So, this is a good place to take a short detour and look at what we mean by the term.

According to the *Shorter Oxford English Dictionary* (2007), philosophy is the 'love, study, or pursuit (through argument and reason) of wisdom, truth, or knowledge'. There are different strands of philosophy. These include natural philosophy, moral philosophy and metaphysics, but for our purposes in relation to research, the definition given above is perfectly apt because, as you will come to understand, no matter what type it is, research is about studying and pursuing truth and knowledge – including wisdom – by means of argumentation and reasoning.

So, when you come across the word 'philosophy' in relation to research, you will understand what we are talking about.

To continue, it is important for us to understand these philosophies, or beliefs, when discussing research because they guide and influence researchers on how to conduct research according to the type of research they are undertaking. Although this chapter introduces you to the idea that there are different types of research that the researcher can use, the types of research themselves are explored more fully in chapter 5 as well as in the web program.

To simplify things here, this chapter focuses on the two main types of research that are in frequent use, namely:

- qualitative research; and
- quantitative research.

In this chapter we explore the philosophical assumptions underlying each type and some of their characteristics. By understanding these different perspectives, you will gain a grounding in the issues addressed in the different types of research. To help you understand the assumptions that underlie research, we begin by looking at qualitative research.

Philosophical assumptions of qualitative research

Creswell (1998: 15) defines qualitative research as:

> 'an inquiry process of understanding based on distinct methodological traditions of inquiry that explain a social or human problem. The researcher builds a complex, holistic picture, analyses words, reports detailed views of informants, and conducts the study in a natural setting.'

When you read this definition, you may immediately come to the conclusion that anything to do with research is quite complicated. But as you work through this and subsequent chapters, as well is through the web program, it will all become clear. You do, however, need to read a definition like the one above and at first try to grasp the substance of what is written rather than worrying about individual words.

We can help you to make sense of what Creswell is saying by giving an example of what this means in a healthcare context.

A researcher undertakes a study to examine the experiences of patients who, in the last 12 months, have used respite facilities (facilities that can be used by chronic and/or seriously ill patients for short-term stays in order to give their carers a break, or respite – e.g. a hospice) provided by their local NHS provider. The researcher may choose to interview the patients in order to ask them about their views on the service. The interviews may take place in the patient's home or at the respite facility. The perspectives provided by the patients are later analysed and a report is produced which gives a picture of the views of the patients who have used the service. So, you can see that qualitative research aims to explore and understand individuals' beliefs, experiences, behaviour and attitudes. It is therefore not a unitary (single) approach to research, but embraces a number of approaches which have their roots in interpretative methodologies (these occur in research studies in which the data are interpreted in order to give meaning to them and hence to the participants' lives). Such methodologies seek to explain and critique an understanding of the socially constructed nature of 'facts' through which individuals or groups make sense of their everyday lives and interactions (Parahoo 2006). In other words, what occurs in people's lives are usually situated within their, and possibly others', families/local/national/international societies, whichever or whatever that might be. There is a social element to everything we do and experience, and this is reflected in our attitudes to, experiences of, confrontations with and perceptions of society and our place in it.

There are five main philosophical assumptions (Guba & Lincoln 1988, Cresswell, 1998) about research, and the explanation of these assumptions has different interpretations in qualitative and quantitative research. Table 2.1 sets out the different philosophical assumptions and how they can be used in qualitative research (after Cresswell 1998). These philosophical assumptions are characteristic of all qualitative inquiries.

To Do

Table 2.1 summarises the philosophical assumptions of qualitative research and examples of its use in practice. To help you to understand them better, write in your own words some simple definitions of the five assumptions referred to in the table. We have given an example of the first one:

Ontological assumption = what is reality (for the individual person)?

Table 2.1 Philosophical assumptions of qualitative research and examples of its use in practice.

Assumption	Question posed by assumption	Features of the assumption	How the assumptions are used in qualitative research
Ontological	What is reality?	Reality is subjective, has multiple voices because of the views of the different participants; variables are complex; insider's point of view (known as emic).	The researcher uses words/ phrases provided by the participants of the study.
Epistemological	What is the relationship between the researcher and the topic under investigation?	Researcher may be closely involved in the study, but explains strategies used to create a distance between the researcher and the study. Empathy is a feature of this type research.	The researcher conducts the investigation in the natural setting with the participants, thus gets a thorough perspective of the participants' routine. Behaviour is influenced by the setting in which it occurs.

Table 2.1   (*Continued*)

Assumption	Question posed by assumption	Features of the assumption	How the assumptions are used in qualitative research
Axiological	What role do personal values play in the investigation?	Researchers acknowledge that their personal values may become entwined in the research, thus creating bias.	Researchers discuss how their own values may influence the discussion and include this, as well as the participants' values.
Rhetorical	What is the type of language used?	Researchers use the participants' language, which may be informal.	Researchers may write in the first person and use language that typifies qualitative research.
Methodological	How is research conducted?	Researcher study the topic in its natural setting and use inductive logic and a design that have roots in the way the study has developed.	Researchers give a detailed description of the context of the study and its participants; the questions may be revised according to information gleaned from earlier discussions with participants.

(after Cresswell 1998).

Some major characteristics of qualitative research

This is a brief introduction to this type of research study and, as has been stated above, the characteristics of qualitative research are discussed more fully in chapter 5. Patton (2002) succinctly identifies the major characteristics of qualitative research under three strategies:

- design;
- data collection;
- analysis strategies.

These headings are used below to explain the characteristics of qualitative research, and now are briefly discussed.

Design strategies

In qualitative research, ideally:

- Studies are conducted in a natural setting, the purpose being to gain insight and improve our understanding of the topic under discussion by exploring its depth, richness and complexity.
- The design of the study is flexible in order to encapsulate (or include) changes in situations which may develop as the research

takes place. For example, research questions may need to be substantially modified whilst the study is under way. Also, the sample of interviewees may need to be modified. In other words, the research is discovery-oriented – it develops as new data are discovered. This design is also described as emergent and open-ended because there are no closed questions or answers – the development of the design is fluid and dynamic, and theory and understanding of the phenomena emerge as the study progresses.

- The participants have specific knowledge concerning the phenomenon (often because they are the ones living with/experiencing it) and thus they are recruited in order to provide an understanding of the issue within a particular context.

Data collection strategies

Data

We have used the word 'data' quite a lot so far, so now is a good place to explain what we mean, because research can only take place if we can obtain data from someone somewhere.

'Data' is the plural of the Latin word 'datum', so one piece of information should be referred to as a datum. Data are quite simply pieces of information. The word 'data' derives from the past participle of the Latin word 'dare' which means 'to give', therefore data are things that are given – that is, facts and opinions that have been given.

In the field of research, data can consist of numbers, words, pictures or music, etc. that are accepted as they stand. In other words, they are not being interpreted in any way – they just are. Data are thus often seen as the lowest level of object/number/words from which we can derive information and knowledge of a subject, situation or phenomenon.

We can now return to data collection strategies in qualitative research:

- Frequently used data collection methods include observation, interviewing, documents, photographs, videotapes and field notes. These methods allow 'thick description' (Patton 2002) and 'rich information' (Polit & Beck 2004) to be gathered about individuals' experiences and viewpoints (see chapter 5 and the web program). In other words, the topic is examined in depth and so the findings are narrow and deep, as opposed to shallow and wide as is often the case with quantitative research (see chapter 5).
- The emphasis is on the researcher-as-instrument (i.e. just as in quantitative research the instrument for the collection of data might

be an experiment, or an actual measuring instrument, so in qualitative research it is the researcher who is the instrument for the data collection). The researcher is able to get to know the participants, sometimes over a long period of time, and so the researcher's views are also important to understanding the situation being explored, as well as to the views of the participants (see chapter 8 and the web program).

- The reality of the process is fluid, dynamic, situational, context-specific and personal; it is therefore socially constructed (i.e. developed within social boundaries, no matter how narrow or broad these might be).
- The data include words, images and categories, rather than just numerical data. In qualitative research, the data can be collected as words, pictures, physical appearance, gestures or music. Indeed, the whole gamut of human experiences and achievements can elicit data in many forms, including numerical (see chapter 8 and the web program).
- The focus is exploratory and descriptive – it describes and explains a phenomenon/situation how will stop.

Analysis strategies

Once we have obtained our data, we need to do something with them – we have to analyse them so that we can start to make sense of them, and give meaning to our findings and to the phenomenon that we are investigating.

Consequently, with regard to the analysis of data, in qualitative research:

- The researcher searches the data for patterns and themes at an early stage, and uses these to explore the data further within the research study.
- This process is one of ongoing inductive analysis. Inductive analysis is analysis which takes us 'beyond the confines of our current evidence or knowledge to conclusions about the unknown' (Sloman & Lagnado 2005: 95). We use inductive analysis in order to ascribe properties or relations to one or more things/people based on a number of observations or experiences. From this we can formulate theories based on recurring patterns of phenomena. This procedure/analysis is a common process in qualitative research because it allows the observer/researcher to become immersed in a group. The researcher obtains initial answers from the participants, and from these formulates further questions throughout research study. These theories can continue to change depending on what the observer finds out from the participants or wants to explore.

- Qualitative researchers are interested in making sense of the data – they are interested in the ways in which people try to make sense of their personal worlds and in the societies that they find themselves in, whether that be their family, work, healthcare setting, hobby or sport.
- Understandings and generalisations are primarily grounded (based) in the data that are collected and analysed. It may then be necessary to organise further studies, or access further studies by other researchers, in order to verify what has been theorised from your initial study.
- To help with the verification of the analysis and theories generated from a piece of qualitative research, some researchers send transcripts of the interviews and focus group discussions to the participants and invite their comments on their analysis of the data in order to seek their opinions of the analysis and interpretations.
- Some researchers distinguish their own 'voices' from those of the participants and some inform readers of their position or status within the research. For example, they may be in a managerial position and are researching the staff they employ. This relationship should be highlighted in the research and how they have overcome the potential conflict explained to the reader.
- The aim of data analysis is to focus on the relationships of the phenomenon under investigation in order that meaningful insights are provided.
- In reporting their findings, researchers present the diverse voices of the interviewees through stories, narratives and quotations.

In summary, we can see that qualitative researchers are:

- Interested in the process of the phenomena. 'Phenomena' is the plural of 'phenomenon', and means 'happenings', events, occurrences. They may be physical, social, psychological or even metaphysical – but let us not worry about that at this stage.
- Interested in the meanings that people give to their world.
- The primary instrument for data collection and analysis.
- Able to produce a descriptive picture of events in the participants' own language/pictures.
- Able to build concepts and develop theories using an inductive process (see the second bullet point above for an explanation of induction in research).

Philosophical assumptions of quantitative research

Having briefly explored qualitative research, we can now turn our attention to the second major research paradigm – quantitative research.

Paradigm

A paradigm is 'a pattern that is followed', and in philosophy is a way of viewing the world which underlies theories and methodologies within a specialty at any given time.

Consequently, in research, we tend to use the term paradigm to describe the major research methodologies, i.e.

quantitative paradigm = quantitative methodology

qualitative paradigm = qualitative methodology.

You will quickly learn that quantitative research is very different from qualitative research in many ways, although their basic aim is the same – to uncover the truth that underlies a phenomenon.

Quantitative research usually seeks to establish causal relationships (i.e. does 'A' cause 'B'? e.g. does smoking cause lung cancer?) between two or more variables – in simple terms a variable is anything that can vary (see chapters 8 and 9, and the web program) – using statistical methods to test the strength and significance of the relationship (Parahoo 2006). Quantitative research is rooted in natural science. In research, natural science includes those methodologies that use scientific methods in order to study and investigate problems and phenomena.

Quantitative research provides data that can be translated into numbers, for example, the National Census, which collects information about people and households in England and Wales and provides a wide variety of information from national to neighbourhood level.

So we can see that quantitative research is an approach which measures phenomena rather than just describing them (although it should be pointed out that there is also a field of descriptive quantitative research, discussed in chapter 5) and produces numerical values which can be analysed statistically. In a healthcare context, randomised controlled trials, cohort studies and case-control studies are quantitative (see chapters 5 and 7).

In terms of sample size, quantitative research is undertaken on a larger scale when compared with qualitative research, which though operating on a smaller scale produces much deeper and richer data, and helps to provide accurate statistical data from which generalisations to whole populations can be made (see chapter 5). As with qualitative research, it is a systematic scientific investigation, but one that uses totally different research strategies and tools.

Also, it should be stressed that the philosophical assumptions and questions relating to the assumptions are basically the same as in qualitative research, although there are important differences regarding the features of the assumptions and how they are used in research. These are shown in Table 2.2.

Table 2.2   Philosophical assumptions of quantitative research and examples of its use in practice.

Assumption	Question posed by assumption	Features of the assumption	How the assumptions are used in quantitative research
Ontological	What is reality?	There is an objective reality; outsider's point of view (known as etic*)	Begins with a hypothesis and/or theories
Epistemological	What is the relationship between the researcher and the topic under investigation?	The researcher does not have any personal effect on what is being researched; detachment and impartiality	The research may be conducted in a laboratory; formal instruments are used; experimentation may be part of the process. The researcher is independent of what is being studied
Axiological	What role do personal values play in the investigation?	The researcher's personal values do not form part of the investigation; objective portrayal	The study is value-free and unbiased
Rhetorical	What type of language is used?	The language is formal and based on set definitions; reduces data to numerical indices	Abstract language used in reporting the results of the study. Scientific theory may be used to explain the data
Methodological	How is research conducted?	Cause and effect; generalisations are made, which lead to prediction, explanation and understanding; the methods are reliable and valid	All aspects of the study are designed before data are collected. Manipulation and control of variables may be used in the study, components of the study are analysed and deductive analysis is conducted

After Creswell (1998).
*An 'etic' account is a description of a behaviour or belief by an observer which can be applied to other cultures (i.e. it is culturally neutral). This is the opposite of an 'emic' account which is a description of a behaviour or belief which is perceived as being meaningful (either consciously or unconsciously) by and to a person within his or her own culture.

Some major characteristics of quantitative research

Just as we found with qualitative research, there are some major characteristics that identify and underlie quantitative research, namely:

Design strategies

In quantitative research:

- Studies are conducted in a highly controlled setting (e.g. a laboratory). The purpose behind this is to provide reliable data which can be generalised to a given population; it also establishes cause-and-effect events (e.g. smoking and lung cancer). This is very different from qualitative research which, as you now know, usually takes place in a natural setting (e.g. the home).

- The design of the study is clearly set out before the study begins and categories are identified before the work starts, unlike qualitative research, which often develops as the research progresses
- Participants in the study have an equal chance of being selected. This is known as random selection (see chapters 5 and 7).

Data collection strategies

In quantitative research:

- These strategies include structured questionnaires incorporating mainly closed questions (i.e. those that require a simple number or a yes/no answer) as opposed to qualitative research, which usually uses open-ended questions from which discussion can proceed.
- Research questions are concerned with how many, or the strength of association between, variables.
- The structured research instruments allow for all respondents to be asked the same questions in a context-free environment, unlike qualitative research in which the context is crucial to an understanding of a phenomenon.
- The sample size is calculated by statisticians using mathematical methods to establish how many participants will be needed from a given population in order to achieve findings with an acceptable degree of accuracy; this does not apply to a qualitative study (see chapter 7). In other words, researchers try to obtain a sample size which will give results with, say, a 95% confidence interval (see chapter 9). This means that if the study is repeated 100 times, in 95 cases you would get the same results. There is therefore a +/−5% margin of error (do not worry if this seems beyond you at the moment; after you have worked through the web program and chapter 9, you will have no problems understanding it).
- The nature of the data can be converted into numbers. With qualitative research, data can be numbers, but are more likely to be in the form of words and pictures.
- The focus of the study is generalisability, prediction and causal explanations; in other words, the focus is objective. With qualitative research, the focus is totally different, because it is expected to be subjective, and the results can only be applied to the people who took part in the research study.

Analysis strategies

In quantitative research:

- Data analysis techniques are determined by the research objectives, questions or hypotheses and the level of measurements achieved by the research instruments (Burns & Grove 2003) (see chapter 9 and the web program).
- Analysis techniques include descriptive and inferential analysis (i.e. inferring from the results to a larger population with the same problem) (see chapter 9).
- The researcher reduces and organises the data to give them meaning.
- The interpretation of the research outcomes involves examining the results from the data analysis in order to:
  - reach conclusions;
  - explore the significance of the findings;
  - consider the implications for healthcare;
  - generalise the results;
  - make suggestions for further studies.

Summary

In summary, quantitative researchers:

- Aim to classify features, count them and construct and use statistical approaches to explain them. In other words, they strive to determine the relationship between one thing (an independent variable) and another (the dependent or outcome variable in a population).
- Design the study clearly before they begin the research process.
- Know in advance what they are looking for (although they may not always find it).
- Use tools such as questionnaires or equipment (e.g. measurements produced by blood pressure equipment) to collect numerical data.
- Know how to test a hypothesis (see chapters 3 and 9).
- Are detached from the study under investigation. This last point is very difficult for a qualitative researcher, who often is part of the study (see chapter 5).

Using mixed methods in research

Finally, it is important to let you know that some research cannot be clearly classified as either quantitative or qualitative. Rather it is a mix of the two, using methods such as data collection and analysis from both.

Mixed-methods research (also known as 'triangulation' – see chapter 5) is a way of undertaking research that employs more than one type of research method – usually a combination of qualitative and quantitative methods – and is used mainly to understand a problem. In triangulation, qualitative methods are used to explore new areas prior to implementing a population-based survey or to explain, in greater detail, an aspect arising from the quantitative aspect of the study.

Rossman & Wilson (1991) give three main reasons for linking qualitative and quantitative data:

1. To confirm or corroborate the data by triangulation.
2. To elaborate or develop analysis, thus providing richer information.
3. To stimulate new ways of thinking by providing different viewpoints.

However, researchers need to consider the complementary differences of each approach, the purpose of their use in the study and how they will be used, that is:

- Will they be of equal status?
- Will they be used separately?
- How will they be sequenced in the study?

(Miles & Huberman 1994).

There are long-standing theoretical and conceptual debates about the merits of the two approaches, with some authors taking a firm view on one or another. For example, Kerlinger believes that there is no such thing as qualitative research – everything is either 1 or 0, (quoted in Miles & Huberman 1994: 40); whereas Campbell (1974) posits that all research ultimately has a qualitative grounding (quoted ibid.).

In sum, a qualitative approach can be of benefit in quantitative research during the data collection phase by making access to and collection of data easier; and during the analysis phase by assisting in interpreting, clarifying and illustrating quantitative finding.

Scenario

Below are three research questions/problems. You wish to undertake some research studies in order to answer them, but have to decide which research methodology will be best suited to answer the question.

1. What is the quality of life of adult patients who have survived a bone marrow transplant for leukaemia?

2. How do the height and weight of children with cystic fibrosis in the UK compare with the standard height and weight of children in the UK?
3. How do homeless adolescents cope with ill health?

Which of the three methodologies discussed in this chapter would best allow you to answer these questions? Give reasons for your decisions based on what you have learned in this chapter.

When you have worked through this scenario, look at our answers/suggestions at they end of this chapter.

Summary

This chapter has introduced you to the more important aspects of qualitative and quantitative research paradigms. You will have noticed that both approaches to research have the same assumption headings. However, when you examine them in more depth, you can see that their functions are very different.

In this chapter, we have noted that some research studies employ both types of research. These basic foundations of research will be revisited throughout this book and are explored in detail in subsequent chapters, particularly in chapter 5.

Activity

Note a topic area in which you are interested, using a single paradigm.

Using the assumptions, write as much as you can about how you envisage the research will take place. Keep this activity as you may wish to return to it later as you work through the book to track your knowledge and progress.

References

Burns N. & Grove S. K. (2003) *Understanding nursing research* (3rd edition). Philadelphia: Saunders.

Creswell J. W. (1998) *Qualitative inquiry and research design: choosing among five traditions*. London: Sage.

Guba E. G. & Lincoln Y. (1988) Do inquiry paradigms imply inquiry methodologies? In D. M. Fetterman (Ed.) *Qualitative approaches to evaluation in education* (pp 89–115). New York: Praeger.

Miles M. B. & Huberman A. M. (1994) *Qualitative data analysis: an expanded sourcebook* (2nd edition). London: Sage.

Parahoo K. (2006) *Nursing research: principles, process and issues*. Basingstoke: Palgrave Macmillan.

Patton M. (2002) *Qualitative research and evaluation methods.* Thousand Oaks, CA: Sage.

Polit D. & Beck C. (2004) *Nursing research: principles and methods* (7th edition). Philadelphia: Lippincott Williams & Wilkins.

Rossman G. & Wilson, B. (1991) Numbers and words revisited: being 'shamelessly eclectic'. *Evaluation Review* **9**(**5**): 627–643.

Sloman S. A. & Lagnado D. A. (2005) The problem of Induction. In K. Holyoak & A. Morrison (Eds.) *The Cambridge handbook of thinking and reasoning* (pp. 95–116). New York: Cambridge University Press.

Stevenson A. (Ed.) (2007) *Shorter Oxford English dictionary on historical principles* (6th. edition), Oxford: Oxford University Press.

Scenario – Possible suggestions/answers

Remember, these are your three potential research studies:

1. What is the quality of life of adult patients who have survived a bone marrow transplant for leukaemia?
2. How does the height and weight of children with cystic fibrosis in the UK compare with the standard height and weight of children in the UK?
3. How do homeless adolescents cope with ill health?

1. What is the quality of life of adult patients who have survived a bone marrow transplant for leukaemia?

You may well have thought that the question would best be answered within the qualitative paradigm, and you could be right. The reason that you probably thought of it as a qualitative research study is that 'quality of life' is, as the name suggests, a qualitative concept – which, of course, it is.

However, it could also fit within a triangulation piece of research. Why? Well, what goes to make up our quality of life? Yes – it is partly to do with how we feel at any one time, and that is subjective. But there are also some objective data that we could collect. For example:

- incidences of ill health;
- physical and mental disabilities;
- employment, or unemployment;
- marital status;
- finances;

and so on.

No doubt you can think of others.

So, these we can enumerate, and therefore some of the data could be quantitative, whilst those to do with feelings could be qualitative. Consequently, if you want to get a full picture of quality of life and what factors may influence it, then you may want to use a mixed methodology – or triangulation. However, if we just wanted to look at people's perceptions of their quality of life, then we would use a qualitative paradigm to investigate this.

2. How does the height and weight of children with cystic fibrosis in the UK compare with the standard height and weight of children in the UK?

I think that you probably all got this right because it is totally unambiguous. We want to compare statistics – height and weight – so we would use a quantitative paradigm. We would measure the weights and heights of a sample of children with cystic fibrosis, work out the means of these weights and heights, then compare these with the means of the weights and heights of the national population by comparing with the height and weight centile charts. We can then manipulate the statistics to our heart's content. Simple, isn't it?

3. How do homeless adolescents cope with ill health?

Coping is often seen as a qualitative attribute, and so we would probably use a qualitative paradigm to help us to answer this question – perhaps using interviews and observations.

A note of caution though: we might (as with the first problem) want to look at some quantitative data to help us to understand how these adolescents cope with ill health – the number of times they have been ill, whom they consulted/saw about their ill health and how often, and what factors contributed to their ill health as well as what types of ill health they are suffering from. In this case you might want to investigate this using a triangulation study.

However, a qualitative study would suffice, depending on what you wish to investigate.

Conclusions

After working through this scenario, you have should have learned two facts:

1. It is not always easy to be dogmatic about which research paradigm you will use to investigate a problem you are interested in – this demonstrates the importance of narrowing down your investigation and making your question lie within very narrow parameters, so that there can be no ambiguity, as the second problem demonstrates so well because it is clear what you want to investigate and how you will go about it.
2. Your research proposal is crucial to producing good research because it is whilst developing and writing your proposal that

you narrow down your question and focus of investigation as well as ensuring that you have chosen the correct research methodology to use in order to answer your question or solve your problem.

These three potential research studies demonstrate why your research proposal is important and why this book and web program are so focused on learning how to write a good, relevant and valid research proposal.

The Research Proposal: Developing the Research Question

Introduction

We continue with the research process by addressing the research question or problem to be investigated. From now on, the chapters are linked very closely to the web program, and so to get the most out of this book you should read the relevant section of the web program alongside the chapters.

In this chapter we concentrate on the development of a research question. This is followed by a discussion of types of questions.

Developing the research question

It is impossible to overstate just how important it is for you to start your research journey with a firm, sensible, clear, concise, relevant and achievable research question or problem. That is the focus of this chapter.

Important features of a good question include the following. It should:

- **be about one issue** – if you attempt to undertake more than one, then your research will become very complicated and you will lose rigour and credibility with it;
- **be clear and concise** – if your research question is not, you and everybody who comes into contact with, or reads, your research will struggle to make sense of what you are attempting to investigate;
- **address an important, controversial and/or an unresolved issue** – there is no point in repeating research, unless you are attempting to verify previous research;

- **be feasible within a specified time-frame** – you need to work out how much time you have available for your research and tailor your question so that you know that it can be answered within that period;
- **be adequately resourced** – you need to know that you have the resources to enable you to finish your research. Therefore, your research question has to be developed so that you are sure from the outset that you have all the resources necessary to carry out the research.

However, at this point we need to stress that, in developing your research question and undertaking your research, of crucial importance is your interest or, better, your passion, in the topic. So, it is essential that your research is focused on an area or subject where you are confident that your interest/passion will not flag during the often long periods you will need to devote to it.

How do you go about developing a research question? You may be very familiar with the area in which you wish to undertake research, but how do you narrow it down to just one question? Table 3.1 (below) offers an example of where to begin. Initially, it is advisable to formulate several questions related to your research area so that you can choose the one that best suits your interests and circumstances. This could be seen as the first stage in the hour glass notion of research identified in Figure 3.1, where you begin with broad questions. Your question may be derived from the patient's problem or condition.

To Do

At this stage, as an introduction to the concept of writing research questions, you may wish to develop questions of interest from your own practice using Table 3.1 as a guide.

Questions arising from the patient's condition

So, after this brief diversion, we can now return to the first stage of research, namely writing a research question.

This stage consists of:

1. The different types of questions.
2. How to find the answers to your questions.

Let us step back from the focus on the research question to discuss briefly what a research study consists of. Developing and undertaking a research study is an eight-step process:

1. Think of an area/topic in which you are interested – discuss this with your colleagues.
2. Begin with broad questions.
3. From these broad questions you can narrow the scope of the question by focusing on determining what you want to find out.
4. Once you have your question, you can then carry out the research.
5. Research consists of observing what happens – whether with experiments or people. Observing is another term for collecting data because data are collected by means of observation of what is happening or what you are finding out during this stage of the research study.
6. Analyse the data – try to organise your data in order to make sense of them.
7. Arrive at conclusions – decide what the research has shown/proved/identified.
8. Finally, go back to your original question to see if your findings have answered it.

If the research study has not answered your original research question, what should you do? What has gone wrong?
Possible reasons include the following:

- The wrong question was asked in the first instance (see below).
- The wrong sample was chosen (see chapter 7).
- The wrong data were collected, using the wrong tool(s) for collecting them (see chapter 8).
- The wrong method of data analysis was chosen, or errors were made in the analysis – particularly of statistics (see chapter 9).
- Quite simply, you chose the wrong research methodology to underpin your research question (see chapter 5).

Whilst reading this book and working through the web program, refer to Table 3.1, so that you can keep in the forefront of your mind the process that is involved in research.

Figure 3.1   The hourglass analogy of research.

In order to think about these two stages, let us use as an example an aspect of a patient's condition or treatment.

When nursing a patient it is not unusual for you to consider why the patient is being cared for in a particular way or whether there is an alternative. How would you answer your concern or problem? One of the points that you need to be clear about is the question that you want to ask. This may not be as easy as it sounds, because if you do not ask the right type of question, you will not get the correct answer. Before we continue, you have to be aware that the answer that you receive

Table 3.1 Developing the research question.

Broad topic area	Narrow topic area	Focused topic area	Research question
Men's health	Men and cancer	Men and lung cancer	Is there an association between cigarette smoking and lung cancer?
Men's health	Men and mental health	Men, mental health and cannabis use	What are the mental health effects of cannabis use in men aged 15–25 years?
Computer games	Computer games and violence	Computer games, violence and children	What is the association between computer games and violence in children aged 5–12 years?
Women's health	Teenagers and eating disorders	Teenagers, fashion and eating disorders	What role, if any, does fashion play in the development of eating disorders among teenagers?

from your research study may not be what you expected, or even what you wanted, yet your research may still have been successful. In all cases, however, the answer must be related to the original research question; if not, the research can be deemed to have failed.

Let us take a closer look at the types of questions that may arise during your consideration of a problem you have identified.

Types of question

You will need to decide on the type of information you require as this will help you to formulate the question that needs to be asked.

There are two types of questions: background questions and foreground questions (McKibbon & Marks 2001).

The broad, narrow and focused topic areas can be seen as the first and second stages of the hourglass analogy of research.

1. Background questions

This is the first stage of forming a question, and these background questions allow you to find out more about the patient, problem or condition under investigation. These are questions about:

- Who?
- What?
- When?
- Where?
- Why?
- How?

and are related to the problem.

An example of such a background question is:

• What causes backache?

Note that there are no inclusion or exclusion criteria and a search of the literature for this question would produce a large quantity of information that might be helpful in assisting with your focused question(s). Thus, background questions give basic information about the condition and may help you to formulate the specific or foreground questions.

2. Foreground questions

Unlike background questions, foreground questions ask for specific information about managing the patient or problem (McKibbon & Marks 2001).

Foreground questions can be related to:

• **Diagnosis:** this includes selecting the most appropriate diagnostic test or interpreting the results of a particular test.
• **Treatment:** here you may look at what the most effective treatment is, given a particular clinical problem.
• **Harm or aetiology:** this takes us into the realms of what the harmful effects of a particular treatment are and how can they be minimised or reduced.
• **Prognosis:** under this heading, we can look at what the likely course of the disease is in this patient or group of patients.
• **Service redesign:** this type of question is moving away from the individual patient and exploring systems and processes. These types of questions have a profound impact on the individual patient. An example of a possible research question is: is it cost-effective to move the care of patients with chronic respiratory conditions from secondary to primary care?

Sackett et al. (1997) devised a framework which can be used to ask foreground questions:

Patient or Problem, Intervention, Comparative intervention and Outcome (PICO).

In some cases there may be a comparative intervention (i.e. drug trials, where you are comparing a new drug with the status quo treatment), but this is not always the case. Table 3.2 provides an example of how PICO can be used. All this relates to the second stage of the hourglass model (see Figure 3.1), that is, to the narrow question by being more focused on identifying exactly what you want to find out.

It is important at this stage to note that none of the above forms part of the research proposal. Only the final question/problem that you have decided that you want to explore will appear on the research proposal. However, all that we have just been discussing will help you

Table 3.2 Components of foreground questions using PICO.

Component of the clinical question	Patient or patient's problem/ condition	Intervention	Comparative intervention (optional). Is there an alternative treatment to compare with the intervention?	Outcome
Example	In patients with mild hypertension	(do) anti-hypertensive medication	or exercise and diet	make a difference in the reduction of hypertension?
Example	In premature babies with sickle cell trait	what are the current treatments		(in the) management of high temperature and infection?
Example	In acute infection	are topical antibiotics	and a placebo	equally effective to achieve clinical resolution?
Example	When providing care for patients with type-2 diabetes	does standard care when compared with	primary/community care	make a difference to patient outcomes and reduction in cost?

to settle on the question or problem that you wish to explore in your research study, and that is a question or problem that will appear as part of your research proposal (see the web program).

Now you have devised your question, the next step is to locate the sources that are available to arrive at the answer. This forms the second aspect of the questions arising from the patient's condition and is discussed next.

Finding the answers to your questions

A number of resources may be at your disposal. For a start, you could consult a clinical nurse specialist or a nurse consultant, if there are any in your hospital or clinic. You may also consider consulting the 'knowledge manager' or 'information consultant' at your learning resources centre, who may be able to direct you to specialist journals as well as to specialist databases such as Medical Literature On-line (Medline) and Cumulative Index to Nursing and Allied Health Literature (CINAHL) in order to help you to find sources that are relevant to your proposed research study. You should also consider searching the web for information about your topic.

Other sources include:

- Peer-reviewed journals: these include research-based articles. These should provide enough details about the methodology employed so that you can make an informed judgement about the study's validity and the clinical relevance of the findings (see chapter 4 and the web program).
- Government publications: include funded research reports, discussion papers, conference proceedings, government policies and enquiry results.
- Organisations and professional bodies: these often provide free information as well as providing you with further sources of evidence.
- Indexes and abstracts to theses: these are often to be found in the libraries of your local Higher Education Institute or your hospital library; if not, all are available from the British Library.
- Reference collections: on past students' work, dictionaries and encyclopaedias.
- Conference proceedings – check journals which often publish special editions linked to conferences.
- Pharmaceutical company information – to access this, it is useful to get to know your local drug representatives, as well as visiting drug company stands at conferences. These often have copies of research papers linked to their products.
- Discussion and networking groups – sources here include the Internet and local/national nurse/health professional groups (e.g. the Royal College of Nursing).
- Newspapers – however, if possible, do search for the original source of the article.

You may find yourself becoming swamped with information, depending on how much research has been done in the area you are researching. If this is the case, you will need to narrow your search to obtain a manageable number of articles.

When you are reading research articles you will notice that some research studies pose a direct question as shown in Table 3.1 above, but other research studies may make a statement; this is referred to as a hypothesis and forms the discussion of the next section.

Scenario

You are part of a team responsible for adolescents who are receiving palliative care for inoperable cancer. You are concerned with how they feel about living with cancer as they approach adulthood. You wish to do some research in this area, so how would you start writing your research question?

At this stage, you do not have enough information, but the purpose of this scenario is to enable you to become familiar with the steps that you need to take in order to be able to write a research question for a proposed piece of research.

Suggestions are given at the end of this chapter.

Hypothesis

A hypothesis is a statement that predicts what a particular relationship between two or more variables will be (for more information on variables, see chapter 9). Usually, the relationship involves a prediction about a pre-specified outcome. The hypothesis (or statement) is tested by experiment(s) in order to confirm/refute the phenomenon under investigation, and the experiment seeks to prove/disprove the hypothesis/statement. However, it is important that the statement is made explicitly. An example would read thus:

'Individualised patient-centred pre-dialysis education improves dialysis outcomes when compared to standard education programme.'

This statement can also be written as a question:

'Does individualised patient-centred pre-dialysis education improve the dialysis outcomes when compared to standard education programmes?'

Although both statements say the same thing, the first is a hypothesis, whilst the second is a research question. So when do we use a hypothesis and when do we use a research question? The simple answer is that if the research involves an actual experiment, then you require a hypothesis, because the purpose of the experiment is to prove/disprove the statement, but you cannot prove/disprove a question, you can only answer it.

As with all hypotheses, this hypothesis contains two types of variables: one independent the other dependent. The independent variable can be controlled by the researcher, whilst the dependent variable cannot be controlled by the researcher – in other words, it is independent of the researcher. All this might seem a little complex, so perhaps it is a good time to have brief look at variables (these are discussed in more detail in chapter 9 and the web program). More information on hypotheses can be found in chapter 5 and the web program.

Variables

As the term suggests, a variable is something that varies (changes) and can be described in measurable terms. Burns & Grove (2005: 97) state that 'variables are qualities, properties or characteristics of persons, things or situations that change or vary'.

Variables can be measured quantitatively, for example, height, weight or age; or, they can be described qualitatively, for example, ethnicity, religion or political affiliation. We shall discuss three types of variables in this section, namely:

- independent variables;
- dependent variables;
- extraneous variables.

Independent and dependent variables

An independent variable is something that can be changed or manipulated by the researcher, whilst a dependent variable is the characteristic or object that changes. We can measure the changes that occur in/with the dependent variable after it has been affected by the independent variable.

Example
Let us assume that we have seen or heard that a study has indicated that drinking a specified amount of caffeinated coffee increases the heart rate. The reason that we can be certain that the specified amount of caffeinated coffee that is drunk increases heart rate is that a controlled study had been undertaken in which a prescribed amount of caffeinated coffee was given to selected participants, whilst no coffee was given to a similar (control) group.

- In this situation the factor that can be altered by the researcher is whether or not to give caffeinated coffee and how much to give; in other words, caffeinated coffee is the independent variable.
- The dependent variable is what we can observe as a result of altering the independent variable – in this case, it is whether or not the heart rate increases.
- The alteration in the heart rate is the outcome of the experiment.

So, an independent variable is one that influences the dependent variable, and is measurable and quantifiable.

The influence of the independent variable can be positive, negative or neutral.

To find out if there is a relationship between the independent and dependent variables we can manipulate the independent variable.

Extraneous variables

Extraneous variables may have an unwanted influence on your study as they are beyond the controls that we have in our study. Examples of extraneous variables include:

- age;
- gender;
- ethnicity;
- time of day;
- lighting.

Researchers try to identify and control extraneous variables so that they do not intervene in the understanding of the effects of the dependent and independent variables.

Reflection

Now that we have had a brief look at variables (see also chapter 9 and the web program) let us return to the example given above of whether or not individualised patient-centred pre-dialysis education improves dialysis outcomes when compared to standard education programme.

In this example, which is the independent variable and which is the dependent variable, and why?

Answer

In this example, the independent variable is *individualised patient-centred pre-dialysis education*; in other words, the researcher can alter this during the experiment, whilst the dependent variable is the one that can be observed or measured; in this case, it is *dialysis outcomes*.

Why?

Individualised patient-centred pre-dialysis education is the independent variable, because we can choose whether or not to offer this education. Alternatively, we can alter the type and amount of education that we give – in other words, we can play around with it. Dialysis outcomes, on the other hand, are the dependent variable because we cannot alter them other than by altering the independent variable, i.e. the education. Any changes in the dialysis outcomes are dependent on the education (the independent variable). Note that we have not mentioned anything about extraneous variables, but these may include gender and age, as well as the experience of dialysis. We might also at some stage want to include some of these extraneous variables in another research study in which we compare the success of patient-centred pre-dialysis education in men as compared to women.

So, to summarise, a hypothesis is a prediction of what the researcher expects will happen in the research study and is generally linked to an underlying theory. The research study may be exploratory in order to develop specific assumptions or predictions that can be tested in future research.

We now turn to the different types of research questions that you may come across when reading research studies, and what you may need to consider for your own research proposal.

Types of research questions

Three types of research questions are discussed in this section, namely:

* descriptive research questions;
* relational research questions;
* causal research questions.

To Do

After you had read this section, work out which types of research studies you have come across in the literature or in practice. For example, can you think of any that were descriptive, relational or causal research studies?

Also, look at the research question/hypothesis of these research studies. Can you see how the research question/hypothesis dictates the research methodology of the study?

This is something to think about as you work through this chapter and the accompanying web program, and then attempt at the end of the chapter. You may find it helpful to take notes as you work through this chapter and the web program.

Descriptive

Descriptive research (Houser 2008) aims to provide a description of what causes an event. It answers questions relating to:

- Who?
- What?
- When?
- Where?
- How?

Descriptive research may be quantitative or qualitative. In quantitative descriptive research the aim is to describe the data and characteristics about the phenomena under study but does not provide the reason for the situation, whereas a qualitative descriptive research study might provide the answers. An example of descriptive research is discussing/describing opinions from interested parties (whether professional or lay) about levels of health service provision in a given area. This type of research can be answered using quantitative or qualitative research methods or as a combination of the two (triangulation).

We usually think of quantitative research as being concerned with statistics, but some quantitative research does not include statistics. For example, whilst the methods used in descriptive research may include statistical surveys, they may also include sampling and interviews (see chapters 5 and 7 and the web program). Some descriptive research is exploratory because the key aim of exploratory research is to discover general information about the research topic. Semi-structured interviews are a particularly suitable method to elicit participants' views about the topic (see chapter 8). However, the results of this type of research may indicate that a more structured format is necessary in order to provide or complement the exploratory research.

You can probably see now that the main difference between descriptive statistical research and descriptive exploratory research lies in the research design, not in the actual purpose of the research.

Relational

Relational research looks at the relationship between two or more variables (Polit & Beck 2004), for example:

- the percentage of men and women with positive attitudes about the introduction of polyclinics in primary health care; or
- the percentage of men with depression compared with women.

In these two examples, the relationship between gender and positive attitudes (the first example) and gender and depression (the second example) are examined, and quantitative or fixed design research can address these questions because it is all down to statistics. A fixed design research study refers to something that we have already discussed: that the structure of quantitative research is usually determined before the study begins, unlike much qualitative research, which is ongoing and can change during the research study (and hence is known as a flexible research design study).

Causal

When we use a causal research question (e.g. does a particular factor cause a particular disease as in the smoking/lung cancer equation?), the design of the study examines whether one variable (or more) significantly alters the outcome of another. In this type of research we are looking at the causes of any changes that occur and the effects of the changes – a cause-and-effect relationship (Burns & Grove 2005). The variables relating to cause and effect are also known as independent and dependent variables respectively (as noted in the example on dialysis outcomes above).

An example of a causal research question is:

'Does an intervention programme improve patient self-reported well-being?'

In this case, the independent variables may be counselling as opposed to non-counselling.

A quantitative design is suitable for answering this question rather than a qualitative one because, again, it is down to statistics. However, if we want to know how the intervention programme improves patient self-reported well-being, then we would probably need to introduce a qualitative research study.

All this is just a brief introduction to these different types of research. (Chapter 5 and the web program discuss the subject in more detail.) Now, we can turn our attention to how we can clarify the phrasing we use in the research question.

Clarification of the research question

This is very important because, as we pointed out above, research questions must be clear, concise and unambiguous, otherwise, the research may be muddled and unfocused, lose rigour and not be acceptable as 'fit' research. So, we need to identify the concepts that we refer to in the research question and, if appropriate, express them in a way that can be measured.

In this section, we look at three words/phrases that often cause problems when used as part of a research question or proposal, namely:

- concept;
- research objectives;
- operational definitions.

Concept

A concept is an idea that we use to label a phenomenon – a name we give to things, observations and events. It enables us to link discrete observations and make generalisations. Examples of concepts include:

- ethics;
- social class;
- deviance;
- quality of life;
- depression.

At this stage, you need to be aware of, and understand, that concepts may be concrete or abstract. However, in your research question or proposal you should avoid abstract concepts because the more abstract the concept, the greater the difficulty in achieving clarity and agreement as to its constituent components.

Research objectives

Although not usually included in a research question, but a very important component of the research proposal – and, of course, your research study – the research objectives should underpin your research question and are specifically related to it. Your research objectives (and there are usually more than one, unlike the research aim) may require you to use different methodologies in order to answer fully the research question and satisfactorily conclude your research study.

You may have several research objectives, but not too many, otherwise your research study will become unwieldy and possibly muddled. Like the research question, the research objectives should be expressed clearly and should contain only one aspect of the study. In other words, each research objective should consist of a single statement that is concerned with just one aspect of the research study.

Kumar (2005) emphasises that the research objectives should be communicated in such a way that readers understand immediately what is to be achieved in the research study. This can be achieved by the use of the active voice in communicating your aim. Therefore, objectives are often stated in an action-oriented way using, for example, active words such as:

- to determine;
- to explore;
- to develop;
- to measure.

(Kumar 2005).

The research methods or design that you use to explore your research question will enable these research objectives, or intentions, to be addressed in the study.

Research objectives are more fully explored, using actual examples, in chapter 9 and the web program, under the heading of 'Research outcomes'.

Operational definitions

Operational definitions tell you what to do. For this reason it is important that you are aware of them and understand them and their role in your research study.

As with everything that you do in relation to your research study, it is very important that they are clearly described so that the reader knows from your report how to interpret your concepts in a specific research situation in which you are involved. Thus an operational definition describes how a particular variable is to be measured or how a condition is to be observed or identified (Gray 2004).

For example, we may want to undertake research into the quality of life of people with a long-term condition (e.g. asthma). In this case, we need to define exactly what we mean by 'quality of life' and 'long-term condition' – and even 'asthma' – and how these concepts are to be measured, so that everyone is clear about just what you are referring to (this avoids any confusion and misunderstanding).

To Do

Make a note of what you think 'quality of life 'and 'long-term condition' mean, and then ask a friend to tell you what they think that they mean. Are they more or less the same? If not, perhaps you have not been clear enough in your definition. If necessary, look up these terms in a dictionary.

You also need to be aware that tools for measuring quality of life vary so you need to be clear about which tool you are going to use/ have used so that the characteristic of an individual's experience can be ascertained. In this way, everybody knows what the individual participant in the research study is discussing and not what you think he/she is discussing. Similarly, the determination of long-term condition has specific characteristics and these too need to be made clear.

The clarity of operational definitions assists others who may be involved in your data collection to focus on the same information, thus making the results more reliable. Also, it is important to be certain that your operational definitions are valid; that is to say, they must measure, or accurately describe, your concept (Gray 2004).

When writing an operational definition, choose an explanation that will help with your and others' understanding of the investigation that you are undertaking. When you have finished writing your definition, ask yourself if your explanation will unambiguously inform another researcher what is to be observed or measured. In this way, the reliability and validity of your operational definitions will lend credibility to your findings, whilst at the same time assisting other researchers when they attempt to build on your work.

So you can now see that not only do operational definitions improve the accuracy of communication about the research study, they are also an important communication strategy.

Summary

This chapter has focused on how you can go about developing your question for your research proposal starting with an observed patient problem or an area of interest. This chapter has also addressed how you can begin to answer your question as well as the other research questions you may come across. Finally, the importance of clarifying the variables and other terms in your research proposal and question have been introduced and stressed.

Activity

- Choose a topic for investigation from your work, then:
- Select a paradigm and frame a general research question within this topic area.
- Write a more precise research question such as 'The aim of my research is to ...' (this is your proposed research study).
- Identify the variables and write an explanation of them.

References

Burns N. & Grove S. (2005) *The practice of nursing research: conduct, critique, and utilization*. St Louis, MO: Elsevier.

Gray D. E. (2004) *Doing research in the real world*. London: Sage.

Houser J. (2008) *Nursing research: reading, using and creating evidence*. Sudbury, MA: Jones & Bartlett.

Kumar R. (2005) *Research methodology: a step-by-step guide for beginners*. London: Sage.

McKibbon K. A. & Marks S. (2001) Posing clinical questions: framing the question for scientific enquiry. *AACN Clinical Issues: Advanced Practice in Acute and Critical Care* **12**(4): 477–481.

Polit D. & Beck C. (2004) *Nursing research: principles and methods* (7th edition). Philadelphia: Lippincott Williams & Wilkins.

Sackett D. L., Richardson W. S., Rosenberg W. & Haynes R. B. (1997) *Evidence-based medicine: 'How to practice and teach EBM'*. Edinburgh: Churchill Livingstone.

Scenario – Some suggestions

1. First, you need to ensure that you have the passion and the resources (including the time) to undertake the proposed research study. This may involve discussing it not only with members of your team, but also with your supervisors/ managers.

2. Be realistic about your research skills. Have you ever undertaken research previously, either individually or as part of a research team? If you have not, make sure that you can get the help, advice and support of someone with research experience.

3. Once this has been satisfied, you have to start thinking about your research question. What exactly do you want to know? This is very important because from it will flow everything to do with your research, such as the design, data collection methods and methods of data analysis. You may want to discuss this with other members of the team, who may be able to offer advice on what you need to focus on, and may even be willing to help.

4. Decide whether you are going to have a research question or a hypothesis, as this will determine whether you will undertake a quantitative or a qualitative research study.

5. Brainstorm, either on your own or with others, and write down a list of questions/statements/hypotheses that are connected, however loosely, with your topic.

6. Now look at the published literature (see chapter 4). This will give you a good idea of what has been done and what still needs to be done. It will also give you a good idea of how to set about your research study.

7. Next you can start to narrow down the list of questions/statements/hypotheses that you came up with in step 5 above, until you decide on the exact wording of your question.

This is a simple, step-by-step guide as to how to write a research question or hypothesis. You may not be able to do this at this moment, but after you have read chapters 4 and 5, and have worked through the appropriate sections of the web program, you should be ready to write a research question.

The Research Proposal: Searching and Reviewing the Literature

Introduction

If you have been working through the accompanying web program, you will now have your research question (an actual one or a virtual one) and included it as part of your research proposal. Now that you know what you are going to explore, you need to check if anyone has done something similar and, if so, what their findings are, as this will have an impact on your own research. After all, you do not want to find yourself repeating what someone has already done. In order to discover what has been researched and published, you have to review it in order to assess its value to your research study.

This chapter provides a guide to the principles of searching and reviewing the research literature.

- It introduces you to the hierarchy of evidence which will assist you in deciding the level and merit of the evidence.
- Conducting a literature search can be a lengthy and complex process; however, the time and effort that you expend on this is well worth the investment (Hart 1998). Undertaking a good, sound and relevant literature search and review of that literature demands an organised and systematic approach, so it is very important to keep detailed records of the searches made and the information found. Figure 4.1 provides guidance on searching the literature.
- Later, this chapter introduces you to the steps you need to take in appraising and reviewing the literature that you find.
- The chapter concludes with an activity for you to undertake.

Steps in searching the literature

To help you to understand this chapter, you may wish to use the question that you developed for the activity at the end of chapter 3. You should work through the procedures using your own question.

The flow diagram depicted in Figure 4.1 below takes you through the steps you need to undertake in order to identify and access the relevant published (and other) literature. When you read the next section, you will appreciate that searching the literature is very similar to researching your research question. There is a very good reason for this – you generally need to have undertaken a literature search in

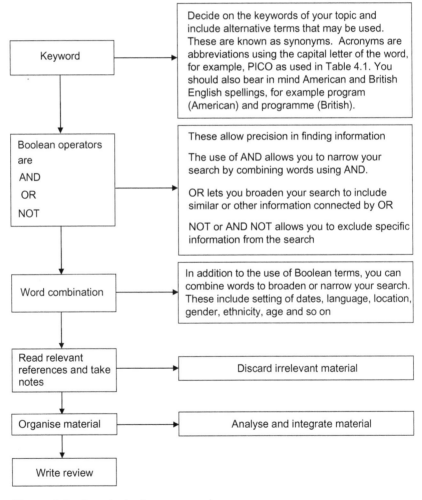

Figure 4.1 Steps in the literature search.
Adapted from Hart (1998), Burns & Grove (2003), Polit & Beck (2004).

order to finalise your research question. So, finalising your research question and undertaking a literature search are simultaneous tasks that you need to carry out when writing a research proposal.

There are many sources that you can turn to in order to undertake a literature search and these are listed below (see also chapter 3).

Sources of literature for reviewing

Specialist databases:

Medical Literature On-line (Medline)
Cumulative Index to Nursing and Allied Health Literature (CINAHL).

The Internet (World Wide Web).
Other sources:

- Peer-reviewed journals: include research-based articles in their publication range.
- Government publications: include funded research reports, discussion papers, conference proceedings, government policies and enquiry results.
- Organisations and professional bodies.
- Indexes and abstracts to theses.
- Reference collections: on past students' work, dictionaries.
- Conference proceedings.
- Pharmaceutical company information.
- Discussion and networking groups.
- Newspapers.

How to undertake a literature search

In undertaking a literature search, you will quickly become aware that there is a large – almost overwhelming – body of literature and other resources, both published and unpublished, you can call on for background information and evidence of relevance to your proposed research study.

When you come to search the literature, the first things that you need to have to hand are 'key words' – words that encapsulate what your research is about. For example, let us suppose that you are going to undertake research into the incidence and causes of falls in the elderly. So, all your key words will need to be linked to the concept of falls in the elderly. Your key words will therefore comprise:

Falls
Elderly

These are the words that you will put into your database (see chapter 3).

We also have to consider synonyms. These are words/phrases that have identical or very similar meanings For example, a synonym for 'falls' that you might wish to consider is 'tumbles'. Why is this important? Well, there may be some literature discussing falls in the elderly that does not use the word 'falls', but rather talks about tumbles in the elderly, so if you only enter the word 'falls' in your database, these papers will be missed. Consequently, you need to think about synonyms for all the terms that you entered into the database and enter these as well.

To Do

Make a list of synonyms for 'elderly'.
   Tip – make sure you have a good thesaurus to hand.

As well as synonyms, you may want to note alternative spellings and acronyms for use in your search.

As mentioned above, you may find there is a mass of information available, although this does depend on how much research has been done in the area you are searching. If you find that there is so much information that you cannot access or assess it all, you will need to narrow your search to obtain a manageable number of articles. We shall return to this later in this chapter when we look at inclusion and exclusion criteria. But for the moment, we are still trying to access as much information as possible, and to help in this, rather than do one search for 'falls', and then a second search for 'tumbles', followed by a third for 'elderly', and perhaps yet another search for 'aged' (a synonym for elderly), we can combine them by using 'Boolean operators'. These are terms such as 'AND', 'OR', 'NOT' which are inserted between our keywords and synonyms.

For example, if we are looking for literature to do with falls in the elderly (but excluding the elderly who suffer a fall because of a stroke), we could insert into our database 'falls OR tumbles AND elderly OR aged NOT strokes'. This will give us all the literature that includes the first four terms, but excludes 'stroke'. Try this combination using the CINAHL database. You will be surprised at the huge number of positive results you get (these are also known as 'hits').

You can combine words without Boolean operators (see Figure 4.1), but this is not usually as effective.

You can also refine your search by reviewing the literature in relation to some of the main themes pertinent to your topic. For example, if you are looking for literature about hypertension, you will need to bear in mind a definition of mild hypertension. You may wish to use the British Hypertensive Society's guidelines or any other suitable definition. You may also want to specify which type of medication you would like to find evidence about. These should be noted.

If, as is quite probable, you receive thousands of hits, then you have to find some way of reducing the number. So, you need to set parameters, such as by having inclusion and exclusion criteria.

Inclusion criteria

Inclusion criteria are characteristics that are essential to the problem under scrutiny (Polit & Beck 2004). They are sometimes referred to as eligibility criteria; in other words, the sample population must possess the characteristics. Examples of inclusion or eligibility criteria include:

- appropriate age groups (e.g. for our example, you may want to have an inclusion criterion that includes only those over the age of 75 years);
- Language (e.g. English);
- location (e.g. Europe, the UK, England, Manchester);
- period (e.g. 2000–10);
- (possibly) evidence-based medicine.

The inclusion criteria of evidence-based medicine will mean that the results of the search will be limited to articles reviewed in databases such as Health Technology Assessment (HTA), Cochrane Database of Systematic Reviews (CDSR) and Databases of Abstracts of Reviews of Effectiveness (DARE). DARE complements the CDSR by providing a selection of quality assessed reviews in those subjects where there is currently no Cochrane review (Greenhalgh 1997, Polit & Beck 2008).

Exclusion criteria

Exclusion criteria are the opposite of inclusion criteria and are characteristics that you specifically do *not* wish to include in your search, such as Caucasians with diabetes if the problem pertains to Afro-Caribbean males with diabetes.

The inclusion and exclusion criteria are important characteristics of a research study as they have implications for both the interpretation and generalisability of the findings (Polit & Beck 2008).

Having obtained the literature, you will need to decide on the relevance of the material found. This can be done by assessing it using a hierarchy of evidence or by reviewing the literature using the research process.

Hierarchy of evidence

The hierarchy of evidence is an aid that we commonly use to assess the value of the material found, and is used in clinical decision-making

(Table 4.1). Hierarchies of evidence were first used by the Canadian Task Force on the Periodic Health Examination in 1979, and have subsequently been developed and used in assessing the effectiveness of research studies (Canadian Task Force on the Periodic Health Examination 1979, Sackett 1986, Cook et al. 1995, Guyatt et al. 1995, Petticrew & Roberts 2003). Thus, the hierarchy of evidence allows research-based evidence to be graded according to their design, is ranked in order of decreasing internal validity (National Health Service for Reviews and Dissemination 1996) and indicates the confidence decision- and policy-makers can have in their findings. However, the hierarchy of evidence remains contentious when applied to health promotion and public health (Petticrew & Roberts 2003).

Briefly, the hierarchical levels of evidence are shown in Table 4.1. (See chapter 5 for more information on these types of research studies and other evidence-based studies.)

There is much unresolved controversy about the kind of evidence that is most relevant to practice – particularly nursing practice and other health professional practice, with the exception of doctors (although many doctors are now seeing the value of 'lower-level' evidence within the sphere of caring for patients and clients). Although there is an undeniable need for quantitative research, this approach is not suitable for many issues encountered in nursing practice (Polit & Beck 2008). Patients' views about healthcare are not always quantifiable – for example, their experience of living with a long-term condition, the effects of treatment or their choice of treatment. These views need to be considered when delivering healthcare when the concept of a hierarchy of evidence is often problematic when appraising the evidence for social or public health interventions. Indeed, the involvement of patients and

Table 4.1 Hierarchy of evidence.

Level	Evidence	
1.	A	Systematic reviews/meta-analyses
	B	Randomised control trials (RCTs)
	C	Experimental designs
2.	A	Case control studies
	B	Cohort control studies
3.	A	Consensus conference
	B	Expert opinion
	C	Observational study
	D	Other types of study, e.g. interviews, local audits
	E	Quasi-experimental, qualitative design
4.		Personal communication

their views are actively encouraged in all nursing and other health professional research projects these days. These issues cannot be addressed appropriately in a quantitative study; a qualitative approach is suitable as this way of conducting research focuses on the meanings and understandings of people's experiences (Burns & Grove 2003).

Another way of demonstrating the hierarchy of evidence is by means of a triangle (Figure 4.2), with the systematic reviews at the top because they are considered to be the strongest evidence, whilst personal communication is considered to be the weakest evidence and so is placed at the bottom. However, although contentious, it may be possible to argue that in terms of healthcare, the hierarchy of evidence triangle should be inverted (turned upside down) because personal communication and qualitative care are concerned with patient care from the patients' point of view, and therefore this evidence should be placed at the apex. In this scenario, objectivity does not apply to the perceptions that patients and other service users (e.g. family members) have of the care given by a healthcare professionals and healthcare organisations.

This is highly subjective, but it is something for you to consider when undertaking your evaluation of the literature you have found. (The triangle follows the classifications found in Table 4.1.)

Another way of deciding on the worth of the material is by reviewing and/or appraising the evidence guided by a systematic process. A

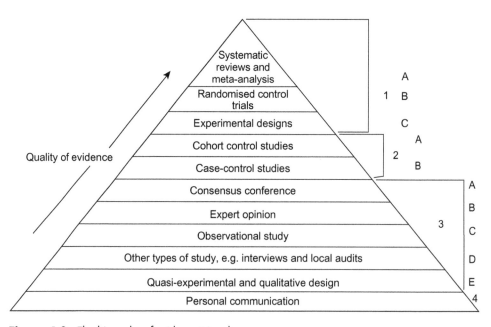

Figure 4.2 The hierarchy of evidence triangle.

Table 4.2   An example of the hierarchy of evidence.
(Source: Booth, A. and O'Rourke, A., Hierarchy of Evidence In: Systematic Reviews: What are they and why are they useful? [Online Module]. University of Sheffield, 1998. Available at: http://www.shef.ac.uk/scharr/ir/units/systrev/hierarchy.htm)

Rank	Methodology	Description
1	Systematic reviews and meta-analyses	**Systematic review**: review of a body of data that uses explicit methods to locate primary studies, and explicit criteria to assess their quality. **Meta-analysis**: A statistical analysis that combines/integrates the results of several independent clinical trials considered by the analyst to be 'combinable', usually to the level of reanalysing the original data, also sometimes called **pooling, quantitative synthesis**. Both are sometimes called **overviews**.
2	**Randomised controlled trials** (finer distinctions may be drawn within this group based on statistical parameters such as confidence intervals)	Individuals are randomly allocated to a control group or a group that receives a specific intervention. In other respects the two groups are identical for any significant variables. They are followed up for specific end points.
3	**Cohort studies**	Groups are selected on the basis of their exposure to a particular agent and followed up for specific outcomes.
4	**Case-control studies**	'Cases' with the condition are matched with 'controls' without it, and a retrospective analysis used to look for differences between the two groups.
5	**Cross-sectional surveys**	Survey or interview of a sample of the population of interest at one point in time
6	**Case reports**	A report based on a single patient or subject; sometimes collected into a short series
7	**Expert opinion**	A consensus of experience from 'the good and the great'
8	**Anecdotal**	Something your friend told you after a meeting

number of factors are important when adopting this process and these are considered next.

Reviewing the literature

This is linked to the Literature section of the web program.

When undertaking research it is important to know what has been written about the topic you wish to investigate by undertaking a literature review. A literature review critically summarises the current knowledge in the area under investigation, identifying the strengths and weaknesses of previous research and knowledge. It provides the context within which you can place your own study (Hart 1998).

Undertaking a literature review requires developing a complex set of skills through practice. This means that you are planning your own research study and organising your time-line (your plan of how much time you can give to the research and how it is to be divided into the various aspects of the study). You will need to allocate enough time to obtain and read the relevant literature and assess its quality. By reading and assessing different studies, you will begin to gain an impression of the important aspects of your proposed topic. These include:

- identifying data sources other researchers have used;
- the style of writing;
- identifying the relationship between concepts in your area of study;
- ideas for further consideration;
- how you can avoid repeating other researchers' errors as well as duplicating previous work.

In addition, you will begin to develop your own reading strategy, as well as your own planning and writing strategies (Hart 1998).

Undertaking a comprehensive review of the literature is particularly important because it:

- provides you with an up-to-date understanding of the subject and its significance to practice;
- identifies the methods used in previous research and therefore ones that you could possibly use – or avoid using – in your own research study.
- helps you to formulate potential research topics, questions and the future direction of your investigation;
- provides you with a basis on which your subsequent research findings can be compared (Gray 2004).

You may also be able to identify the significant personalities in your area of interest – the leaders in the field who have undertaken and published exceptional research in this field, on whom, perhaps, you could 'bounce' your ideas.

Also from the literature you can begin to find out whether any diverse or conflicting viewpoints exist, as well as the aspects of the topic under investigation that have produced significant discussion. Any conflicting viewpoints may arise from differing interpretations of various theories within the same topic. You need to be aware of these interpretations as well as the arguments supporting the theories in order to assess their value and make up your own mind about their merit, relevance and importance, particularly with regard to your proposed research topic and study. All of this will enable you to begin to develop some general explanations for observed variations in behaviour or phenomena that you may be able to elicit/identify in your own research study.

Steps in reviewing the literature

Previously, you have been shown how to identify and obtain the relevant literature – relevant, that is, to your proposed study and to the topic in general. Having obtained this, the next step is to review this literature.

There are a number of ways in which the literature can be reviewed. An important task for the reviewer is to summarise the research papers and to identify and discuss the main studies that have been published in your field of interest. A number of writers (e.g. Grbich 1999, Burns & Grove 2003, Polit & Beck 2008) suggest that a review of the literature can be divided into several sections. The subdivisions discussed here are an adaptation of ideas and writings from these authors. Using the subdivisions and considering the points suggested will assist in this activity. However, you are going to have to understand each report as a whole in order to get a sense of what it is about. These divisions are like the individual bricks in a wall or the single steps in a journey – they are only a part of the picture. It is important to appreciate the wall or the journey as a total experience; the bricks/steps are a way of allowing you to do this.

The structure of the report

- Is the organisation of the report logical? Does it make sense/is it understandable?
- Does the report follow a sequence of steps of the process of research, such as these?
    - Introduction
    - Identification of the research problem
    - Planning the research study
    - Data collection methods
    - Data analysis methods
    - Results
    - Discussion of the study and its results
    - Conclusions obtained from the study
    - Recommendation as a result of the findings from the study.

You need to appreciate that the way in which a report is organised may vary from one researcher to the next. However, in all cases, the organisation should be logical. It should begin with a clear identification of what is to be studied and how, and should end with a summary or conclusion recommending further study or application. You should bear in mind that the various professional journals may require a different layout, but the key issue is that it is presented as a logical progression. So, let us identify and discuss these steps ourselves.

A research report should comprise the following:

The abstract

The abstract of a research paper or report should be presented in a short, coherent, concise paragraph. Therefore, the first question that we have to ask is just that – is it presented concisely? You then need to ask yourself – and answer – the following questions about the abstract:

- What was studied?
- How was it studied?
- How was the sample selected?
- How were the data analysed?
- What are the main findings of the research?

The abstract is very important because it provides a summary of the question and of the most important findings of the study. It outlines how these differ from those of previous studies and gives some indication of the methodology used. It is usually about 200–300 words long, depending on the journals' guidelines or the thesis format of the relevant university. The abstract provides the reader with an overview of what the research has found. However, perhaps its main purpose – and therefore importance – is to capture the readers' attention and make them want to read the whole paper. The abstract is the first part of a research paper that is accessed and read. If it is badly written or does not include the relevant facts, then that might be all that is read, as the readers may lose interest because they do not think that the paper is relevant to them.

The introduction

Now we can move on to the introduction to the research study. This serves to explain why and how the research problem was defined in a particular way. In other words, it should include the rationale for undertaking the research study in the first instance. It should also critically review the published literature that the researcher has reviewed, pointing out any limitations in their findings, methodology or theoretical interpretation. In addition, it provides a pathway to the methodology section by clarifying the need for research to be undertaken in the chosen topic, especially with regards to the methodology and techniques that have been selected to investigate the research question.

The problem statement/purpose of the research

The introduction should be followed by a statement and discussion of the problem that the researcher has investigated in the study (see also chapter 3 and the web program).

In this section, you should consider whether:

- the general problem has been properly introduced and stated;
- the problem under investigation has been substantiated (supported by the evidence) with adequate discussion of the background to the problem and the need for the study;

- the general problem has been narrowed down to a specific research problem or to a problem that contains relevant sub-problems as appropriate;
- if it is an experimental quantitative research study, that the hypothesis directly answer the research problem;
- if it is any other type of research study, that the research question directly addresses the problem identified.

The literature review and theoretical rationale for the study

Now we come to the author's own literature review. In a review of previous literature (including a theoretical rationale for the study to take place) you should aim to consider whether this section is relevant, clearly written, well organised and up-to-date, and whether the reliability of the methods and data collection has been addressed. Your reasons should be substantiated.

- Was there a sufficient review of the literature and the theoretical rationale associated with the previous research to assure you that the author(s) considered a broad spectrum of all the possibilities there were for investigating the present research problem?
- Is it clear how the study will extend previous research findings?

Note that a full report on a research study or an academic thesis requires an extensive literature review, whilst in a journal article/paper the author will usually cite the *principal* pieces of work that are relevant to the study in hand.

Methodology

The methodology section should fully inform readers of the research paper/article of the step-by-step processes that were undertaken in conducting the study (see chapter 5 and the web program).

In this section, you should consider the appropriateness of the research methods chosen, including:

- the sampling approach;
- the data collection methods;
- the validity and reliability of the observations or measurements.

In order to help you to understand this section of a research paper, it is important that you consider the following subheadings and questions under each heading. This will help in providing you with such information.

The population and sample (see chapter 7 and the web program)

Ask yourself the following questions:

- Is the study population-specific enough so that it is clear to which population the findings can be generalised – that is, have the

researchers defined their population and is it closely linked to the topic being investigated?
- Is the study sample representative of the population defined?
- Would it be possible for you or others to replicate the study population?
- Is the method of sample selection appropriate?
- Was any bias introduced by this method? (see Sica's definition in the box below).
- Is the sample size appropriate and how is it substantiated?
    - Is it large enough for a quantitative research study?
    - Are the statistics significant?
    - Is the rationale for the size of the sample given and is it adequate?
    - Is the method of determining the sample size stated?
    - Is it adequate for a qualitative research and is the rationale given?

Bias

'Bias is a form of systematic error that can affect scientific investigations and distort the measurement process. A biased study loses validity in relation to the degree of the bias. While some study designs are more prone to bias, its presence is universal. It is difficult or even impossible to eliminate bias completely. In the process of attempting to do so, new bias may be introduced or a study may be rendered less generalisable. Therefore, the goals are to minimise bias and for both investigators and readers to comprehend its residual effects, limiting misinterpretation and misuse of data' (Sica 2006: 780).

Instrumentation – method of collecting data (see chapter 8 and the web program)

- Are the data collection methods used appropriate to the study?
- Did they obtain the data that the researcher was searching for in order to answer the research question/hypothesis?
- Has the author discussed the validity and reliability of the instruments used within the context of the research study?

The procedure for data collection (see chapter 8 and the web program)

- Were steps taken to control extraneous variables? (see chapter 3 for a discussion on variables).
- Are the collection methods used replicable in another similar piece of research?

Ethical considerations to be addressed (see chapter 6 and the web program)
These are the questions should be asking yourself whilst reading the section on ethics in the research paper.

- Were the rights of the subjects/participants involved in the research addressed?
- Has the researcher included in the report any discussion of ethical considerations?
- Is there a discussion of the impact of any ethical problems on the merit of the study and the well-being of the subjects?
- Has the researcher presented any evidence to indicate that the rights of the study's subjects/participants have been protected? (e.g. is there a discussion of informed consent with examples?)
- Are the steps that were introduced to protect subjects/participants discussed and are they appropriate?
- Has the researcher discussed any violations of ethical principles that occurred and made suggestions as to how these could have been avoided?

Critiquing the ethics of research studies
Polit et al. (2001) provide useful points to bear in mind when critiquing the ethics of research studies:

- Was any coercion or undue influence used in recruiting participants?
- Were vulnerable groups included?
- Were participants deceived in any way?
- Was the study fully explained to the participants?
- Were appropriate consent procedures adhered to?
- Was privacy fully ensured?
- Did the benefits outweigh the risks?
- Was the study approved and monitored by an ethics committee?
- Was the reporting of the results accurate and unbiased (e.g. were any data omitted or changed to fit the findings)?
- Did they change the hypothesis?
- Was there an acknowledgment of any financial support?
- Did they reveal any conflicts of interest?

(Polit et al. 2001).

It should be noted that due to space restrictions, research reports frequently do not provide readers with detailed information concerning adherence to ethical principles. This does not necessarily mean that adherence did not take place.

The pilot study (see chapter 6)
Ask yourself the following questions:

- Was a pilot study undertaken?
- Were any changes made following the pilot study? If not, why not? If there were, were these discussed and rationalised, and evidence produced for the changes?

Analysis of data (see chapter 9 and the web program)
When we look at the section on data analysis, we need to remember that data and their analyses differ according to whether the research undertaken uses a qualitative design or a quantitative design, so at the outset we have to make that distinction clear. So, depending on the type of research design being reported, ask yourself the following questions, as appropriate:

- Was the analysis of the data clear and is it related to the hypothesis or research question?
- Have the researchers made it clear which statistical methods they used and what values were obtained. Have they given a rationale for their choice of statistical test?
- Is there a statement of whether or not the data support the hypothesis?
- Has a thorough examination of each hypothesis, including the use of appropriate statistical analysis and the decision to accept or reject the hypothesis, been included?
- Have the researchers indicated whether the data have answered the research question?
- Have the researchers explained how and why the data collected and analysed have answered the research question?
- Have the researchers shown how the data have given rise to 'themes' that will answer the research question?
- Have the researchers provided a comprehensive discussion of the data?
- Have the researchers given an explanation of how missing data (if any) were handled?
- Have experts been used to assist in the analysis of the data?
- Has the analysis of the data been verified by an expert?

Discussion (see chapter 10)
The discussion is an extremely important part of a research paper because this is where all the threads are drawn together and the results/findings are discussed and put into context. So ask yourself the following questions:

- Have the researchers critically presented a discussion of the research study, particularly the analysis and the findings?
- If it is a quantitative research study, can the findings be generalised?
- Have the researchers made sense of the findings within the context of the study?

Conclusions and limitations

At the end of the research paper, ask yourself the following questions:

- Have the researchers related their findings to the theoretical proposition underlying the study?
- Have the researchers identified any methodological problems?
- Have the researchers over-generalised, or are they specific about what the results have shown?
- Are the implications of the findings for practice identified? If not, have the researchers discussed why not?
- Are there any suggestions for further research? Usually, all good research should leave the reader wanting more. Good research can often leave more questions than have been answered in the research study.

References and bibliography

If a reference and bibliography section is included, ask yourself the following questions:

- Are all the references cited relevant to the study? If not, has a rationale been given for their inclusion?
- Do the references and bibliography reflect the review of the literature?
- Do they relate to the search for and/or development of valid and reliable instruments/methodology?
- Are any important references missing?

There is a lot here to consider, but it is worthwhile taking the time to review the literature thoroughly before undertaking your own research study, as it will make your task of producing a research proposal much easier.

Hart (1998) warns that when reading or undertaking a review, you should be aware of your own value judgements and try to avoid personal, destructive criticisms. 'Critique' and negative 'criticism' are not the same thing, although they do both derive from the same root word, because, while a criticism is negative, a critique looks fairly at a piece of work and seeks to highlight the positive as well as the negative. So, do be fair and try to understand what the researchers are trying to say.

Having undertaken the literature review related to your own research proposal, you may be in a position to consider the most productive methodology for your research, given the time and resources that you have available. This forms the focus of chapter 5.

Scenario

Now it is your turn to try your hand at critiquing some research.

In the box below you will find an excerpt from the literature review in a research report on the needs of people with cancer and their families that was undertaken by one of the authors with a colleague. Note that this is a research report rather than a research paper. Therefore, as had been mentioned above, it is much fuller than would be expected in a research paper, which is really a summary of a research report.

As your intention is to undertake research into 'the stresses on families of coping with a dying family member', you need to undertake a literature review of the material you have obtained, and this is one such piece. Read the excerpt and then write a critique of it using the questions above that are relevant to the study. Bear in mind that it is only a small excerpt, but it will give you practice in this very important skill.

Mention has already been made of Rokach et al.'s (2007) study into the 'loneliness experience' of the dying and of those who care for them. Family caregivers may feel helpless in the face of the diagnosis, the symptoms and treatment, and the anticipated death of someone whom they love and whose lives they have shared intimately for several years. Caring for a dying person can be emotionally and physically unbearable for family members, and yet they are expected to take on this role without any previous training or insight. Consequently this can create considerable strain on the family caregivers, and may affect their work, family life and social relationships, making them more isolated, lonely, and dependent upon the company of someone who is in pain and distressed. Rainer & McMurry (2002: 1421) put the situation so succinctly when they wrote 'the physical changes that accompany the dying of a loved one can be difficult to watch and often impossible to understand. Adding the mental, spiritual, social and emotional adjustments may make this event overwhelming'.

As Hanson (2004) points out, several studies have acknowledged the stressful nature of this 'emotional work' that the carers have to cope with and manage. In the concept of management, Hanson notes that this involves managing the emotions of their relative who has cancer, as well as managing their own perceptions and feelings, including guilt, anger, sadness, and one that has been mentioned above, namely 'uncertainty' (Kellett & Manion 1999, Scott et al. 2001, Soothill et al. 2001, Wennman-Larsen & Tishelman 2002, Thomas et al. 2002).

Hanson (2004) uses the work of Andershed to discuss three key themes that are important to the family caregiver (Andershed 1999, Andershed & Ternestedt 2001). These three key themes are those of knowing, being, and doing. The three themes have been identified as relating to the principal support needs of families of terminally ill people.

Commencing with knowing, this is concerned about all relevant family members being informed about a range of issues, just as much as the family member who is terminally ill. It is very important that carers know about their family member's disease, diagnosis, prognosis, accompanying symptoms, treatment and care, as well as ongoing health status (Andershed & Ternestedt 2001). This is important because family members need to be able to plan for the remaining length of time that they have with their family member who has cancer (Steinhauser et al. 2000a, Steinhauser et al. 2000b). This also allows an opportunity to consider the death that they know is to come, including discussing personal fears about the death and the future afterwards (Payne et al. 1997). In addition, it is important that family members have knowledge about what is expected of them in their new caring role, and how to cope with everyday life living with someone who is terminally ill and the crises that may crop up during their everyday lives (Rose 1999, Scott et al. 2001). This includes knowing what services are available to help them in their roles, and also, just as important, how to access them (Sheldon 1997).

The second of these themes, namely 'being' is concerned with being with one's relative, to spend time together and to be close to one another (Hanson 2004). This consists of emotion on psychosocial elements, such as sharing the illness and struggle together (Kellett & Manion 1999), as well as more practical elements, such as being able to be with them rather than at work (Andershed 1999). Hanson (2004) notes that 'being' is also concerned very much with the abilities of the family and the person with cancer to be able to talk openly about their feelings together, although as both Rose et al. (1997) and Thomas et al. (2002) point out, it is often difficult for them to be able to share these feelings, particularly about death and the loneliness and fears for the future following the death. However, Wennman-Larsen & Tishelman (2002) note that various studies have shown a number of family carers regret not being able to express their feelings openly with their dying partner.

Soothill et al. (2001), also within this theme of 'being', stress the importance of a carer being able to have time for himself or herself, and also to be able to spend time with others, rather than just with a family member with cancer) in order to reduce their feelings of isolation and loneliness. This brings up the need for respite care services to help to reduce the burden of the family caregivers and to give them regular breaks from their caring duties, so that they themselves do not suffer physically, mentally, and emotionally to such an extent that they are unable to function properly as a carer, and ultimately following their bereavement. Scott (2001), referring to Maslow's hierarchy of needs, stresses the importance of the family caregiver being able to ensure (or given the opportunity) basic requirements for rest, relaxation and sleep as an essential step to allowing them to be able to deal with their emotions such as anxiety, fear and uncertainty, as well as the needs of self-esteem and self-actualisation (Hanson 2004).

There are no right or wrong answers. You should simply review the piece using what you have learnt in this chapter.

Summary

The discussion presented in this chapter offers guidance to help you to undertake a literature review that will underpin your own practice. A literature review is essential for any research that you may undertake; it is also a useful skill to have in relation to your job. Undertaking a literature review will provide you with up-to-date knowledge of your area. Practitioners must make every effort to keep abreast with the latest research data pertaining to their area, bearing in mind that they are accountable for their practice. Key points to remember about the literature review include the theory, the methodology and the gaps in the literature.

Activity

Using a research paper that you have found from you literature search of your question/topic, attempt to review as much of the paper as possible by using the process outlined above in 'Steps in reviewing the literature'.

References

Burns N. & Grove S. K. (2003) *Understanding nursing research* (3rd edition). Philadelphia: Saunders.

Canadian Task Force on the Periodic Health Examination (1979) The periodic health examination. *Canadian Medical Association Journal* **121**: 1193–1254.

Cook D. J., Guyatt G. H. et al. (1995) Clinical recommendations using level of evidence for antithrombotic agents. *Chest* **108**: 227s–230s.

Gray D. E. (2004) *Doing research in the real world*. London: Sage.

Grbich C. (1999) *Qualitative research in health*. London: Sage.

Greenhalgh T. (1997) Papers that summarise other papers (systematic reviews and meta-analyses). *British Medical Journal* **315**: 672–675.

Guyatt G. H., Sackett D. L. et al. (1995) Users' guide to the medical literature: 1X. A method for grading healthcare recommendations. *Journal of the American Medical Association* **274**: 1800–1804.

Hart C. (1998) *Doing a literature review: releasing the social science research imagination*. London: Sage.

National Health Service Centre for Reviews and Dissemination (1996) *Undertaking systematic reviews of research on effectiveness. CRD guidelines for those carrying out or commissioning reviews*. Heslington: University of York.

Petticrew M. & Roberts H. (2003) Evidence, hierarchies and typologies: horses for courses. *Journal of Epidemiology and Community Health* **57**: 527–529. http://jech.bmjjournals.com/cgi/content/ful/57/7/527

Polit D. F. & Beck C. T. (2004) *Nursing research: principles and practice.* Philadelphia: Lippincott, Williams & Wilkins.

Polit D. F. & Beck C. T. (2008) *Generating and assessing evidence for nursing practice* (8th edition). Philadelphia: Lippincott, Williams & Wilkins.

Polit D. F., Beck C. T. & Hungler B. P. (2001) *Essentials of nursing research: Methods, appraisal, and utilization* (5th edition). Philadelphia: Lippincott.

Sackett D. L. (1986) Rules of evidence and clinical recommendations on the use of antithrombotic agents. *Chest* **89**: 2s–3s.

Sackett D. L., Richardson W. S., Rosenberg W. & Haynes R. B. (1997) *Evidence-based medicine: How to practise and teach EBM.* Edinburgh: Churchill Livingstone.

Sica G. T. (2006) Bias in research studies. *Radiology* **238**: 780–789.

The Research Proposal: Research Design

Introduction

Crookes and Davis describe the research design as 'the overall plan of how the researcher intends to implement the project in practice' (2004: 73). In the same vein, Parahoo (1997) talks about research design as a plan within which the researcher details the how, the when and the where of the way data will be collected and analysed during the study.

This chapter introduces, and discusses, the elements that come together to produce a well-designed research proposal, followed by the research study. It is linked to the study design section of the web program.

A proposed research study must be structured in such a way that the results and conclusions are reliable and can be seen to be rigorous. In a well-designed study, the various elements follow one another seamlessly, but the starting point for developing any research design is the selection of a topic and a paradigm. A paradigm is a method, or pattern, by which the topic of the research is explored (this is discussed later in this chapter). Other elements in a research design include:

- the use of previous literature on the topic (chapter 4);
- the purpose statement, which will include questions, objectives and/or hypotheses (chapter 3);
- the ethical issues (chapter 6);
- the proposed participants in the research – the sample (chapter 7);
- the methods of data collection (chapter 8);
- how the data are going to be analysed (chapter 9);
- how the results will be disseminated (chapter 10).

This chapter encompasses and discusses all the elements that make up a good research design.

The focus of a research study

'The heart of every research project is the problem. It is paramount to the success of the research effort. To see the problem with unwavering clarity and to state it in precise and unmistakable terms is the first requirement in the research process' (Leedy & Ormrod 2005: 43).

Before you can start doing any research, you need to select a problem to investigate: this is the focus of your research study – the central concept that you will be examining (Creswell 1994). There is frequently some confusion as to what is a suitable focus for a research study. It is often thought of as solving a problem. However, this is by no means the case. The focus of your research study may well be solving an existing problem, but the focus could also be identifying whether or not there is a problem or, if you know that a problem exists, what it actually comprises.

How do you select a problem to be the focus of your study? This involves asking the right questions in the right way and/or communicating with others who are familiar with the area that you wish to explore. It is highly unlikely that the problem you select as a potential focus for your research will be totally unique. Usually, some work will have been carried out on the problem you are interested in, although the aspect of the problem that has been previously investigated may be different. For example, one of the authors undertook a research study into the early hospitalisation of children following bone marrow transplantation for severe combined immune deficiency and the effect of that and of isolation on them and their families. These topics had already been explored in relation to cancer, for example, but this was the first time anyone had looked at these concepts in relation to severe combined immune deficiency. As a result discoveries were made, which were also found to relate the children with cancer and others in a similar situation.

Returning to your need to select a focus for your investigation, this might come about due to:

- something that you have read in a professional journal or book;
- something that you have seen in your professional practice, wherever that might be sited;
- something that somebody has mentioned as being of concern and/or interest – this could be another professional (healthcare or other), a patient/client, a family member of a patient/client or someone totally unconnected with your work (e.g. a friend or even a chance meeting with a stranger);
- your general interest in the area;
- an inspirational thought – never discount inspiration.

Once you have selected your general focus, you have to narrow it down to something much more specific so that you arrive at a particular problem that you wish to investigate (this is the same process that you came across in chapter 3). To help you narrow down the parameters (limits or boundaries) of your focus, you need to specify what that problem is. Research problems are usually stated in the form of a question, although they can also be stated in the form of a hypothesis (a proposition that is assumed to be fact for the sake of an argument), for example:

Questions

- Why do some patients improve on a particular drug regime, whilst others do not?
- Do families who have a child who has undergone a bone marrow transplant have any psychosocial problems?
- How can we prevent cross-infection in a hospital ward?
- What are the needs of adults dying of cancer?
- What is the safest way of x-raying an infant?
- How best can we improve the quality of life of someone in a wheelchair?
- What is the safest way to transport a neonate with meningitis to a specialist hospital?

Hypothesis

- Smoking causes lung cancer.

Producing a hypothesis/research question

Above, we have considered problems which provide a possible focus for several different research studies. However, these are still quite broad in scope. In order to design a research study to look at a particular focus, we need to refine our question. This we can do by means of a hypothesis or a specific research question.

A **hypothesis** is basically a question that is turned on its head so that it becomes a statement (see also chapter 3). The purpose of a hypothesis is to stimulate experimental research so that you can either prove or disprove the statement that makes up the hypothesis. Thus, if we look at the first four research questions listed above, we can develop the following four hypotheses from each of the questions that describe the particular problem that we wish to investigate. The hypotheses for each of these four problems can now be written as:

- Patients with liver disease who are in hospital will improve when prescribed a particular drug, whilst those patients who are at home and are prescribed the same drug do not improve.
- Families with a child who has undergone a bone marrow transplant suffer from severe psychosocial problems.

- Cross-infection in a hospital ward can be prevented by rigorous hand washing.
- Adults who are terminally ill with cancer need the support of specially trained health professionals.

The researcher then has to come up with an experiment to test these hypotheses and either prove or disprove them.

You can now see that each of these problems has a much narrower focus. This makes it easier for us to design a research study to tackle that particular problem.

> **To Do**
>
> Take the next three research questions in the list of questions above and develop hypotheses (the plural of hypothesis) from them.
>
> Then take the hypotheses in the list above and make a research question out of them.

Null hypothesis

Some researchers are concerned that if we use a hypothesis, we will be predisposed to be favourable to it and that might bias our research study. Consequently, some prefer to use a **null hypothesis**. In effect, this is a negative statement, such as:

- Smoking does not cause cancer.

To ensure that there is no positive bias in the research study. It is thought that by introducing a possible negative bias by using a null hypothesis, then if the research does produce a positive result, it is seen as stronger, more rigorous and valid research.

> **To Do**
>
> Now take all the hypotheses that you have come across so far in this chapter and turn them into null hypotheses.

Research question

Not all research is experimental. Non-experimental research does not require a hypothesis, because in non-experimental research you are not trying to prove or disprove something; rather, you are exploring a problem. This is usually the case in qualitative research as opposed to experimental quantitative research that does require a hypothesis, but it has to be noted that a lot of quantitative research is also non-experimental – for example, research within the category of descriptive quantitative research.

With non-experimental research, whether quantitative or qualitative, we do not use a hypothesis because we are not trying to test something but are investigating a problem. When working within non-experimental research paradigms we often use research questions rather than hypotheses to underpin the research. Research questions are usually more general than hypotheses and so allow for modification and expansion of the elements that make up the research question as the research study develops.

To return to our first four research problems, possible research questions that can be developed from these problems include the following:

- Why do patients in hospital improve when taking drug A, whilst patients at home do not?
- What are the psychosocial results for a family whose child has undergone a bone marrow transplant?
- Will hand washing on its own prevent cross-infection in a hospital ward?
- What do adults terminally ill with cancer perceive the needs to be that can be met by the palliative care services?

In each case, we have narrowed down the initial problem to a question that can provide a specific focus for a research study, and by so doing we have helped to clarify not only what we will be investigating, but how we will be investigating it.

To Do

Now take the remaining research questions from the list and try to clarify and narrow their focus so that you begin to have questions that can be more easily investigated.

So far in this chapter we have discussed the focus of the research study because this is probably the single most important aspect of research design and of research itself. A poor hypothesis/research question can lead to a poor research design and consequently a poor research study, whilst a good hypothesis/research question can lead to good research design and a good research study because all the other elements of the research design and study are dictated by, and come from, the initial hypothesis/research question. As Leedy & Ormrod (2005: 43) state:

'the problem or question is the axis around which the whole research effort revolves. The statement of the problem must first be expressed with the utmost precision; it should then be divided into more manageable subproblems. Such an approach clarifies the goals and directions of the entire research effort.'

Research paradigms

'The design of a study begins with the selection of the topic and paradigm. Paradigms in the human and social sciences help us to understand phenomena' (Creswell 1994: 1).

In research, paradigms are composed of various sets of beliefs and practices that are shared by researchers. These paradigms provide frameworks and processes through which research and investigation can be carried out (Weaver & Olson 2006). Within each paradigm you will find a combination of vocabularies, theories, principles, presuppositions and values related to a particular research inquiry (Bunkers et al. 1996, Weaver & Olson 2006). Weaver & Olson (2006) simplify matters by defining paradigms as being sets of philosophical underpinnings from which specific research approaches flow – for example, in nursing we tend to be concerned with quantitative (or positivist) and qualitative (or naturalistic) methods and approaches to research inquiries. (Research philosophies are explored more fully in chapter 2 so we will not consider them in this chapter.)

However, within these two paradigms, there is a 'rich array of approaches and methods available' (Polit & Hungler 1999: 14), and it is up to the researcher to decide which paradigm, and which approach and method, to use in order to explore the problem. This is where the importance of the research question/hypothesis comes in. The paradigm, including the approach and methodology, is dictated by the initial research question/hypothesis. If the research question/hypothesis does not properly reflect the problem/inquiry, then the methodology could be inadequate or even completely wrong for the research. As a result, either the research will fail or it will be very poor research indeed. In other words, it is important that the research question/hypothesis is first framed and agreed by you, the researcher (and your research team if you are part of one), and then the most appropriate method is chosen by which the question can be answered or the hypothesis proven or not proven. The researcher should 'choose the correct tool to do the job rather than just using the tool and then asking "now what job can I do?"' (Crookes & Davies 2004: 74). In other words, select your topic and then determine your hypothesis or research question. Only then should you decide on the actual research paradigm that will allow you to prepare, and successfully complete, your research study.

We shall explore below the research design in terms of the two paradigms mentioned above, but you need to be aware that there are certain aspects of any research study that are common to all research. These include:

- ethical issues;
- the rigour of the research;
- ensuring that you have the correct sample for your particular research study;
- writing the research report;
- the dissemination of results from your research.

Samples

As you prepare your research proposal, you will need to consider who is going to participate in the study. This is called the sample. A sample is a group of people who have been selected as representatives of a population as a whole. A 'population' (in terms of a research study) consists of the people who may be affected by the phenomenon(a) you are investigating. The sample must be large enough to allow you to investigate fully the phenomenon(a) using the research methodology that you think will best answer the research question/problem/hypothesis.

Different types of sample can be used, according to your research methodology, research question/problems and the aims of your research. These different types of research samples include:

- random samples;
- theoretical samples;
- purposive samples;
- convenience samples;
- snowball samples;
- volunteer samples.

These different types, and how we decide which one to use, are discussed in chapter 7 as well as in the web program.

Next we consider the research design in terms of the two major paradigms used in nursing research – quantitative and qualitative paradigms.

Quantitative research

Quantitative research is the principal method we use when considering scientific investigation in nursing (Burns & Grove 2005). According to Porter & Carter (2000: 19), quantitative research is 'a formal, objective, systematic process for obtaining quantifiable information about the world, presented in numerical form and analysed through the use of statistics'.

We use a quantitative research paradigm to test relationships between phenomena and it is particularly brought into use to examine cause-and-effect relationships (e.g. smoking and cancer, or obesity and type-2 diabetes).

Norbeck (1987) notes that there is a belief among researchers that quantitative research provides a much sounder and more reliable knowledge base for the purposes of guiding nursing practice than does qualitative research because quantitative research is thought to produce 'hard' science involving:

- rigour;
- objectivity;
- control.

Unlike researchers who use qualitative methodologies, quantitative researchers believe that truth is absolute and that there is a single reality that can be defined by careful measurement. Therefore, in order to find this 'objective truth', the researcher must be completely objective. In other words, the researcher's values, feelings and personal perceptions are not allowed to be brought into the measurement of 'reality'. Consequently, quantitative researchers hold that all human behaviour is:

- objective;
- purposeful;
- measurable.

Within the quantitative research paradigm, there are several methodologies that the researcher can use, namely:

- experimental research;
- quasi-experimental research;
- non-experimental research (including descriptive research and correlational research);
- survey research;
- evaluation research.

Experimental research

Experimental research is the type of research that most people think of whenever quantitative research is mentioned (Polit & Hungler 1999). It is the most appropriate and powerful quantitative method for testing cause-and-effect relationships because of its rigorous control of variables and it is considered the gold standard for demonstrating something in a rigorously scientific manner.

Experimental research involves observation, usually to test cause-and-effect relationships between variables under conditions which, as far as possible, are controlled by the researcher. It involves not only scientific observation, but also the manipulation and control of phenomena. According to Porter & Carter (2000), a classic experimental research design involves the selection of subjects (a sample) who are randomly allocated (see below) to either an experimental group, who are exposed to the variable that is the purpose of the study, or a control group, who do not come into contact with the variable, and hence act, as the name implies, as a control within the experiment.

You will come across these types of research studies particularly in relation to trials for new drugs.

Double-blind tests are typically used in drug trials. 'Blinding' means that either the patient or those providing care to the patient do not know whether the patient is in the experimental group or the control group. 'Double-blinding' means that neither the patient nor the caregivers are aware of the group assignment of the patient. The purpose of double-blinding is to ensure that the risk of bias (particularly subconscious bias) from either the patients or the caregivers is avoided.

Randomisation

Note that in quantitative research we think of randomisation when we are looking at the make-up of our sample. Randomisation means that we choose the subjects of the sample randomly. As a result, every individual in a population has an equal chance of being selected for the sample. One of the reasons why we would opt for randomisation (random sampling) is that it helps to eliminate any bias that might distort our findings. We have already mentioned that, in experimental studies, we may use an experimental group and a control group (e.g. when testing a new drug). In this case, subjects would be randomly selected for the study, and then further selection would take place when the subjects selected for the study are randomly assigned to the experimental group or the control group.

Quasi-experimental research

Quasi-experimental research may look very much like true experimental research in that it involves the manipulation of an independent variable, but it is not the same, because quasi-experimental research studies lack one or both of the essential experimental research properties of randomisation and a control group.

The main drawback with quasi-experimental research is that, compared to experimental research, it has a weakness in that it is not possible to deliver cause-and-effect results (Polit & Hungler 1999). In other words, we cannot infer from quasi-experimental research that, for example, doing one thing causes a particular phenomenon.

Descriptive research

This type of research, as its name suggests, describes what exists, but it may also uncover new facts and meanings that were previously not known or apparent.

The purpose of descriptive research is to observe, describe or document aspects of a situation as it naturally occurs (Polit & Hungler 1999). This involves the collection of data that will provide an account or description of individuals, groups or situations. Examples of the types of instruments that we use to obtain data in descriptive studies include questionnaires, interviews (closed questions) and observation (e.g. checklists). There is no experimental manipulation, or indeed any random selection to groups, as there is in experimental research.

The characteristics of individuals and groups such as nurses, patients and families may be the focus of descriptive research. It can provide a knowledge base which can act as a springboard for other types of quantitative research methods.

Correlational research

Correlational research within a quantitative paradigm aims to investigate systematically and explain the nature of the relationship between variables in the real world. Often the quantifiable data (data that we can count) from descriptive studies are analysed in this way. Correlation means to co-relate; in other words, correlational research studies go beyond simply describing what exists and are concerned with systematically investigating relationships between two or more variables of interest – they co-relate (Porter & Carter 2000). Such studies only describe and attempt to explain the nature of relationships that exist; they do not examine causality (i.e. whether one variable causes the other), as is the case in experimental research.

Survey research

According to Polit & Hungler (1999), a survey is used to obtain information from groups (populations). The information so obtained may be concerned with the prevalence, distribution and/or interrelationships between variables within these groups. For example, the UK census comes under the heading of 'survey research'. In this type of research, data collection tools include:

- personal interviews;
- telephone interviews;
- questionnaires.

It should be pointed out, however, that, depending on the problem under investigation, this type of research may be better explored by means of a qualitative paradigm, although there is still a place for quantitative research methodology in survey research. For example, the UK census return report is based mainly on the quantitative paradigm, but more recently it has included elements from the qualitative paradigm, such as detailed, face-to-face surveys that also take place as part of the census data collection.

Evaluation research

This is an 'applied form of research that involves finding out how well a programme, practice, procedure or policy is working' (Polit & Hungler 1999: 201). The aim is to assess/evaluate the success of a particular practice or policy (see also chapter 1).

Examples of this type of research can be seen in various types of analysis/evaluation, including:

- process/implementation analysis;
- outcome analysis;
- impact analysis;
- cost–benefit analysis.

As with the survey research methods, this type of research may best be carried out as a qualitative piece of research, depending on the original research question.

Scenario

You are a researcher who has been commissioned to investigate the incidence of leg ulcers in the under 50 year olds in the catchment area of a Primary Care Trust situated within a city. Because you are going to be investigating the incidence of something – not the causes or experiences – you will base your study within a quantitative paradigm. The question that you have to answer is: which type of quantitative research will you use for your study, and what will be your rationale for choosing this type of research?

Possible suggestions are given on page 107.

Data collection

There is a variety of techniques that can be used to collect data in a quantitative research study (see chapter 8). However, all of them are geared towards numerical collection (i.e. the data are in the form of numbers rather than words or any other media).

Numerical data can be collected by means of:

- observation;
- interviews;
- questionnaires;

- scales;
- physiological measurements.

In quantitative research, the data are collected and recorded systematically, and are then organised so that they can be entered into a computer database (Burns & Grove 2005). However, some of us are old enough to remember doing this using only pen and paper and our brains (later, we were able to turn to the help of very basic calculators). Computers and computer databases are comparative newcomers in the recording and analysis of numerical data, but they are now so sophisticated that if you enter the correct data, the computer will analyse it in seconds (and even represent the findings graphically).

Piloting and pilot studies

If you are planning to undertake quantitative (or even qualitative) research, you really need to consider undertaking a pilot study before attempting the main study. A pilot study is usually preliminary to a main study and as such should follow the design of the main study as closely as possible – or rather, the main study (amended as necessary) should fully follow the pilot study. In addition, the sample should consist of subjects who resemble, as closely as possible, those who will be used in the main study. Another criterion that a pilot study should meet is the extent to which the areas covered or the questions asked by interview or questionnaire measure what they are supposed to measure.

It is not unusual to exclude participants in a pilot study from the main study as they will have been exposed to the intervention or interview protocol and respond differently from those who have not experienced the procedure (Peat et al. 2002). However, in some cases it may not be possible to exclude the pilot participants as the main sample may be too small, particularly where the research has to reach groups such as prisoners and homeless individuals. Holloway (2005) believes that pilot data are of less concern in qualitative research than in quantitative research because in the former, analysis is often ongoing and so including participants from different stages of the study is less crucial, whereas in the latter, the data could be flawed or inaccurate because all data must be rigorously collected from people with the same experiences of the phenomenon, with no extra variances (Peat et al., 2002). The important point is to justify whichever method you choose to adopt.

The reason for running a pilot study is that it serves as a testing ground for your data collection instruments, sample and method of analysis so that if mistakes are made in any part of your research design, it will not be unduly costly in terms of money or time, because you can sort out the problems before you move on to the main study. The intention to undertake a pilot study should be stated in your research proposal because both the ethics and the research and development committees will expect this.

Qualitative research

The second of the two research paradigms that we are going to discuss is qualitative research. Qualitative research is an umbrella term that covers several styles of psychosocial research and draws on a variety of disciplines, among them sociology, anthropology and psychology. However, there are two common elements to these approaches that begin to give some sense to the term 'qualitative research'. These are:

- **A concern with meanings and the way people understand things.** Human activity is seen as a product of symbols and meanings that are used by members of the social group to make sense of things. One of the symbols and meanings that can be analysed is 'text', i.e. the written or spoken word. Other symbols that we can use in qualitative research include drawings and play.
- **A concern with patterns of behaviour.** The focus in terms of patterns of behaviour is on regularities and irregularities in the activities of a social group, such as rituals, traditions and relationships, and the way that these are expressed.

Qualitative data

Qualitative data, whether they are depicted in words, images or any other medium (including, occasionally, numbers), are the product of a process of interpretation. The data only become data when they are used as such. Data do not exist in their own right waiting to be discovered, but are produced by the way they are interpreted and used by researchers. Qualitative research can be part of an information-gathering exercise and useful in its own right, or it can be used as the basis for generating theories. In neither case, however, are its descriptions ever 'pure'; they are always the outcome of researchers' interpretations. Nevertheless, even quantitative research can never be 'pure', because the numerical data have to be interpreted (even if they have been analysed by computer), and all humans are fallible.

Qualitative research methodology

Introduction
We have already mentioned that qualitative research consists of a number of differently developed methods that are best suited to address questions of particular interest. There are, however, some general themes of qualitative research design that apply to all approaches and methodologies. These are:

- Qualitative design is flexible and elastic – it is capable of adjusting to what is being learned during the collection of the data.
- Qualitative design usually involves mixing various methodologies in terms of data collection (e.g. interviews and diaries).

- Qualitative design is focused on understanding a phenomenon or a social setting.
- Qualitative design tends to be holistic; it involves striving for an understanding of the 'whole', rather than just an understanding of a part of the phenomenon that is being studied.
- Qualitative design requires the researcher to become intensely involved in the research study. This can often be over very long periods of time.
- Qualitative design requires the researcher to become the research instrument.
- Qualitative design requires the ongoing analysis of the collected data. This in turn drives both the collection of more data and the formulation of theories as the research progresses.
- Qualitative design forces the researcher to develop a model based on the data collected as opposed to the quantitative researcher who will develop a theory (possibly as an hypothesis) and then collect the data to support/refute the hypothesis.

As mentioned above, there are many different qualitative research methodologies, but we will consider just three methods that are probably the most common qualitative research methodologies nurses use. These are known as:

- ethnography;
- grounded theory;
- phenomenology.

Ethnography (see also the web program)

The qualitative research methodology known as 'ethnography' is built on the social science specialism known as 'anthropology'. Anthropology is the study of humankind, especially of its societies and customs, and the study of the structure and evolution of the human being as an animal – particularly as a social animal.

An ethnographic research study is one that studies people in their natural environment. It is a descriptive account of social life and culture within a defined social system, and is often thought of as 'a portrait of a people'. In effect, it is concerned with a holistic view of a culture, including its shared meanings, patterns and experiences.

The aim of ethnographic research

This involves the description and the interpretation of cultural behaviour. It is culturally specific patterns of behaviour and attitudes that give people a sense of being members of a group and, under certain circumstances, set the guidelines for action.

Ethnography is a description and interpretation of a cultural or social group or system. The aim of the ethnographic researcher is to learn from (rather than study) members of a cultural group. The ethnographic researcher's intention in relation to the members of a particular cultural group is to understand their worldview as they define it.

The ethnographic researcher examines the group's:

- behaviour;
- customs;
- way of life.

The researcher also studies:

- the meanings of behaviour;
- the meanings of language;
- interactions of the culture-sharing group.

An ethnographer will try to define a particular culture by asking questions such as:

- What does it mean to be a member of this group?
- What makes someone an 'insider' and others 'outsiders'?

The ethnographer also tries to make sense of what people are doing by asking:

- What's going on here?
- How does this work?

And the ethnographic researcher hopes to be told about the way the group does things in their society/culture.

Answering these questions requires openness to learning from those who inhabit that culture and a willingness to see everything and suspend premature judgement on what should be selected as data. This quality of openness lies at the heart of ethnography, in its processes, purposes and ethics. Thus, the whole complexity of cultural categories and assumptions and the variety of relationships among them should be examined.

In ethnographic research studies, the researcher is the main instrument of data collection. The researcher must gain acceptance by the group, but at the same time it is crucial that the researcher does not become so involved in the group and individual members of the group that theoretical distance is lost. In other words, the researcher must not lose objective perspective. This is referred to as the management of marginality.

The ethnographic researcher has to fulfil certain roles 'in the field'. These are:

- complete observer;
- observer as participant (observing while participating in group activities);
- participant as observer;
- complete participant.

It is important that the researcher continually undertakes throughout the study:

- reciprocity (mutual actions, or 'give-and-take');
- reflexivity (the ability to reflect on what they see and also their role in the group/society).

When talking about reflexivity in research, you will realise that this is nothing new for nurses and other healthcare professionals, who should be used to reflecting on their work and relationships with patients.

Reflection

Reflective processes are very important to researchers because they help them see the world in alternative ways by enabling them to focus on different aspects of their experiences (Jasper 2003). They are the stages of thoughtful activity that we all need to go through when we consciously decide to explore an experience or reflect on it.

There are basically six fundamental stages of reflective processes. These are:

- Stage 1: selecting a critical incident to reflect upon.
- Stage 2: observing and describing that experience.
- Stage 3: analysing that experience.
- Stage 4: interpreting that experience.
- Stage 5: exploring alternatives.
- Stage 6: framing action.

Any experience we have had can be used as the focus of reflection, but what we choose to reflect on needs to have some significance for us – that is, significance in terms of what we are trying to achieve or the purpose that it is going to serve. These significant experiences or events are often known as **critical incidents**.

Flanagan (1954: 327) defined what is meant by incidents and critical incidents: 'by an incident is meant any observable human activity that is sufficiently complete in itself to permit inferences and predictions to be made about the person performing the act. To be critical, an incident must occur in a situation where the purpose or intent of the act seems fairly clear to the observer and when its consequences are sufficiently definite to leave little doubt concerning its effects.'

So we can see that critical incidents are episodes of experience that have particular meaning to the observer, the practitioner or any other person taking part in them. They may be positive or negative and must be suitable for being described in a concise way (Jasper 2003).

Reflection in research is exactly the same. However, reflexivity operates at different levels in good research. These include:

- the identification of theoretical frameworks within which the researcher is operating;
- the identification of the researcher's own values;
- reflection on how personal feelings may affect the researcher;
- the description of, and reflection on, the methods used in the research;
- the description of, and reflection on, the context within which the research is conducted.

These are what you, as a researcher, will have to familiarise yourself with. The benefit of this is that as you become more adept at using reflection in your research, so your powers of reflection will improve in practice.

Key stages of ethnographic research
There are several key stages involved in ethnographic research that you have to come to terms with. These are:

- The research question – this is usually open-ended rather than closed.
- Participant observation – this involves the researcher thinking about what is going on and observing members of the culture, whilst at the same time being a participant in the many occurrences that take place within that culture. This is a difficult skill to master – you may find your loyalties becoming blurred and divided, and the boundaries of your roles becoming fuzzy.
- Taking field notes – these are the notes the researcher takes as a participant. They are made at the same time as the experience, or the observation made, by the researcher.
- Reflection and the writing up of field notes – during participation, and afterwards, researchers will reflect on what they are experiencing/have experienced and observing/have observed as participants in the culture. Later, they will need to write up the notes that have been made in the field, in order to put them in order and make some sense out of them. This will help the development of further choices in terms of what the researchers will participate in and what further contacts will be made with members of the culture.
- Interviewing – this can be formal in that the researchers will have a number of questions which they ask during a formal interview with one or more members of the group/culture. Alternatively,

interviewing can be informal – in this case, the researchers will interview members of the group or culture as if they were simply talking to them, whilst at the same time having a good idea of the questions that they want to ask.
- Interpretation of interviews – once an interview (whether formal or informal) has taken place, it is imperative that the researcher writes it down, or transcribes it if it has been recorded, before not only the words have been forgotten, but also the gestures and facial expressions that supported the words. The interviews then need to be analysed and interpreted.
- Writing up the ethnographic research – following the research study, it is important that it is written up in journals and/or a book, as well as being presented at conferences.

Samples

Often only relatively small samples are needed for ethnographic research. Larger samples can be unwieldy and much information and data can be missed.

It is important to remember that the ethnographic researcher is normally an outsider as far as the group members are concerned. Therefore, he/she must continually negotiate access to, and acceptance by, the group members throughout the study.

Group members who are important to the researcher in order to gain access and acceptance include:

- Gatekeepers – the people who allow the researcher access to the group and to individual members of the group.
- Key informants – the people on whom the researcher relies for direction and assistance in terms of acceptance by individual members.

The sample is purposive (chosen for the specific purposes of this research study) in that it selects participants (see chapter 7 and the web program).

Data collection

Data collection always takes place in the field. Consequently, an ethnographic researcher needs a good memory because she/he often has to recall what was said, or what was experienced/occurred, at a later time, rather than as it happens (someone standing around writing in a notebook will stand out as 'alien' in any group situation – and will be seen as being outside of the group which is the very antithesis of being an ethnographic researcher).

Data analysis

Data analysis is ongoing throughout the study. It involves progressive focusing on the data to identify and develop themes. By this means, the researcher aims to develop a cultural portrait of the social group that incorporates both the views of the members of that group and the researcher's interpretation of the group and its functioning from a social science perspective.

Advantages/disadvantages
As with all research methodologies, there are inherent advantages and disadvantages. Ethnographic research has many advantages, and these can be summarised as:

- **Direct observation** – the researcher does not rely on second- or even third-hand reporting, but is able to collect data that he/she has experienced or observed at first hand, and therefore knows that there have been no errors (unless he or she has made them).
- **Links with theory** – throughout the research study, the researcher is assessing the material collected and can compare this with existing theories and/or theories that he/she has started out with, amending the theories as the data dictate. Consequently, not only are the theories continually evolving as new data emerge and are analysed and interpreted, but a direct link remains with the ever-evolving theories.
- **Detailed data** – because of the length of time spent with the participants, as well as the close proximity and observations, and any shared experiences, the researcher can obtain very detailed and rich data indeed.
- **Holistic** – the researcher, by being a participant in the group culture over a prolonged period of time, is able to see many facets of the group/culture rather than just one or two parts of it, and therefore is likely to have a much more holistic view of the culture/group.
- **Validity** – because the researcher is directly involved with members of the group and experiencing what they are experiencing (i.e. all data collected are first-hand evidence), the validity of the research and the findings is much more assured than it would be if it was only relying on external observation or other's experiences and reports.
- **Contrast and comparison** – because of the multiple perspectives obtained through an ethnographic research, the researcher will be able to contrast and compare individual accounts and experiences to build up a picture of a group that is both cohesive and diverse.
- **Actor's perceptions** – ethnographic researchers are acting a role by participating in a group or culture, and whilst they cannot place themselves inside the heads of the members of the group that is being studied, they can develop perceptions which can give them glimpses of the lives and experiences of the participants within their culture, which allow them to have some understanding of the participants' lives and experiences.

- **Self-awareness** – becoming members of a group enables research-ers to be aware of themselves and their feelings as members of that group or culture. This allows them to become more aware of the experiences and feelings of the participant members of the group than would be the case if they were observing from a distance.
- **Ecological** – by becoming part of the group, a claim can be made that the research is ecologically sound – the researcher's resources are the group's resources.

However, although there are many advantages associated with eth-nographic research, unfortunately there are also many disadvantages:

- **Time requirement** – a good ethnographic research study requires a huge investment of the researcher's time, because some studies run for years and the researcher needs to be part of the culture or group throughout the study period.
- **Presentation of results** – this can be a problem for the researcher because the results will be diverse as a result of the multiple percep-tions with which the researcher has to deal (along with the research-er's own perceptions). Add to this the length of time (and the possible large number of participants), and collating all the data and results into a coherent presentation or paper can be very difficult.
- **Reliability** – because the researcher in an ethnographic study is often working alone, there may be nobody who can verify the find-ings for reliability.
- **Interviewer effect** – as a member of the group/culture, but at the same time as an outsider, the researcher may affect the findings, as the members of the group will probably want to present themselves and their group/culture in a good light. This is similar to the so-called Hawthorne effect, which is a kind of placebo effect. The name comes from the Hawthorne plant of the Western Electric Corpora-tion where a series of experiments took place in which various environmental conditions (e.g. lighting and working hours) were varied to determine their effects on worker productivity. Regard-less of what changes were made (e.g. improvements in lighting, worsening of conditions), the productivity of the workers increased. It was therefore concluded that knowing that they were part of a study was sufficient to cause them to modify their behaviour. This masks the effect of the variable that is of interest to the researcher (Polit & Hungler 1999).
- **Inhibitions** – These can be generated among the culture/group as a result of the members being observed, often continuously for an extended period of time, and can possibly affect the functioning of the individual and the group, so that it is no longer being true to itself. It could also be the inhibition felt by the researcher, who may be self-conscious at playing a part that is alien to him/her.

- **Safety** – There are safety issues for the researcher to consider when isolated from his/her natural environment and placed in an alien setting with people who may at times become hostile. In addition, the researcher can feel (and indeed be) very isolated from his/her safety network. This danger can be physical, psychological, emotional or social.
- **Invasion of privacy** – There are concerns over the invasion of privacy that can ensue for the members of the group/culture, who, even though they have agreed for the research to go ahead, may not fully realise to what extent their privacy may be threatened both during the study (by the researcher) and afterwards (by society). **Lack of privacy** – there is also a potential problem of lack of privacy for the researcher, particularly after the study has been completed, if members of the group seek the researcher out.
- **Scale** – there can be problems of scale if the group/culture (or sample of the group/culture) is very large as the collection of data and the results may become too complex for the researcher to be able to make sense of the study afterwards. Also, the larger the group, the more time the researcher requires to complete the study.
- **Ethics** – mention has been made above about the risks of lack of privacy, but there are also ethical concerns over the informed consent of the participants. If the researcher wants to avoid the Hawthorne effect (see above), then members of the group/culture should not know that they are taking part in a study, but if they do not know, they cannot give their consent – informed or otherwise. If they give informed consent, then the dynamics of the group may change – possibly irreparably, but certainly for the duration of the research.
- **Access** – there could be problems with gaining access to a particular group or culture, and the approach could be loaded with tensions on both sides. This may cause the researcher to approach only a 'safe' group with whom he/she feels comfortable and so risk diluting the research. Also, the researcher may be dependent on a 'gatekeeper' – someone who can help the researcher gain access to the group or culture and who may bias the results of the research, or who can get so close to the researcher that concerns over safety as well as objectivity can ensue.
- Other concerns
  - The conduct of the study and its results is often dependent on the skill and rigour of the researcher.
  - Replication of the study can be difficult.
  - There are issues of researcher objectivity and reactivity (to the members of the group and to situations encountered within the group).
  - The transferability of findings may be problematic.

- The links to practice and policy-making may not often be easy to make or there may not be direct links, so making it difficult for implementation.
- Obtaining funding for ethnographic research can be difficult.

Conclusion

In this type of research enquiry, developing a theory is a process. As new data emerge, existing hypotheses may prove inadequate.

The researcher's view of what needs to be looked at and reported on may change, and explanations of what is going on may be supplanted by ones that seem a better fit. In other words, emergent design is a distinguishing feature of this methodology.

The object of ethnographic research is to discover the cultural knowledge that people have, how it is employed in social interaction and the consequences such employment may hold. No attempt to generalise the findings beyond the case itself should be made, since statistical random sampling is rarely a feature of ethnographic research. The intention is to achieve understanding of a specific case. However, Hammersley (1992) suggests that empirical generalisation is possible in some cases if 'typicality' of a defined population at a given time can be established. (Empiricism is the theory that knowledge is derived from experience, rather than taught.)

The goal of ethnographic research is to combine the view of the insider with that of an outsider to describe a social setting. For this reason it is a popular approach to social research, and the outcome of the research study is a form of story-telling – vignettes of people's lives and relationships, inner thoughts, feelings and contradictions.

At the end of the study, the ethnographic researcher must ensure that there is proper closure with the group that has been studied, and that relationships with individual members of the group are terminated cleanly, harmoniously and safely.

Overall, ethnography is a method of deep research, involving spending considerable periods of time with a particular community or group of people. It lends itself to the study of some subcultures and institutions, such as drug users, sex workers and the police.

Grounded theory (see also the web program)

Introduction

The second qualitative research methodology that we shall look at is grounded theory. Grounded theory is derived from sociology and was first proposed by Glaser and Strauss in 1967. The main purpose of a grounded theory approach is to begin with data that have been collected in the course of the research study and use these data to develop a theory. A grounded theory study uses a prescribed set of procedures for analysing data and constructing a theoretical model from them.

Although it originated in sociology, it is now used more and more frequently in other areas, among them education, nursing, psychology and social work.

The term 'grounded' in this context refers to the idea that the theory that emerges from the study is derived from, and hence is 'grounded' in, data that have been collected in the field, rather than data that have been found in the research literature.

Grounded theory studies are especially helpful when current theories about the phenomenon are either inadequate or even nonexistent. Typically, a grounded theory research study focuses on a research process (including people's actions and interactions) that is related to a particular topic. The ultimate goal is the development of a theory about that process.

Generally speaking, grounded theory is an approach for looking systematically at (mostly) qualitative data (e.g. transcripts of interviews or protocols of observations) with the aim being to generate theories.

Although grounded theory is often seen as a qualitative method, it is in fact more than that. It combines a specific style of research (or paradigm) with a pragmatic theory of action and with some methodological guidelines. ('Pragmatic' means being concerned with dealing with matters in terms of their practical requirements or consequences.)

The purpose of grounded theory

The purpose of a grounded theory study is to generate, or discover, a theory. Consequently, it is inductively derived (derived from reasoning) from the study of various phenomena. (Inductive means the inference of a general law or theory from particular instances.) Consequently, the theory is discovered, developed and provisionally verified through systematic data collection and analysis of data pertaining to that phenomenon. It is important to remember that you do not begin with a theory and then attempt to prove it. Rather, you begin with an area of study, then allow what is relevant to emerge from the research so that, eventually, this become a theory (or a set of theories).

Concepts

The important concepts in grounded theory are:

- categories;
- codes;
- codings.

The research principle behind grounded theory is neither inductive nor deductive (the inferring of particular instances from a general law or theory, although deductive is meant to be a *guarantee* of the truth of a conclusion, whilst inductive is concerned with the *probable* truth of a conclusion), but combines both by way of abductive reasoning. (Abduction means inference to the best explanation.) It is a method of reasoning in which one chooses the hypothesis that would, if true, best explain the relevant evidence. Abductive reasoning starts from a set of accepted facts and considers from them what is likely to be the best theory that explains these facts.

All this theorising may seem abstruse, but we have included it because it gives you the background to the principle underlying grounded theory research. Still, now we have got the theory out of the way, we can concentrate on the practical aspects. Theorising leads to a research practice where data sampling, data analysis and theory development are not seen as distinct and discrete (separate) stages, but as different steps to be repeated until it is possible to describe and explain the phenomenon that is to be researched (the 'stopping point'). The stopping point is reached when new data do not change the emerging theory any further – it has reached saturation point. We talk about theoretical saturation when no new data emerge from the data collection tools (interviews, questionnaires, observation, diaries) and analysis.

Key analytic assumptions

There are two key analytic assumptions involved in grounded theory, namely:

1. constant comparison;
2. theoretical sampling.

Constant comparison:

- identifies similarities and differences among the emerging categories (the concepts that emerge from the collected data);
- can construct subcategories from concepts that are found in the data;
- ensures a two-way process of building up the themes and also of deconstructing them into smaller units;
- connects categories so that an emerging theory encapsulates the wide variations and complexities of the data.

Whereas in theoretical sampling:

- the researcher involves individuals who are able to contribute to the theory as it evolves;
- sampling begins with the selection of a homogeneous sample of individuals (homogeneous means 'the same');
- once the theory is developing, it consists of selecting and studying a heterogeneous sample to confirm or to refute the conditions under which the theory can hold to be true (heterogeneous means 'different');

- it may also involve the sampling of incidents, records or literature in order to develop the emerging theory;
- sampling of data will continue until saturation is achieved.

So, when we talk about theoretical sampling, we are concerned with:

- the sampling of new cases as the analysis proceeds;
- the process of data collection and data analysis continuing until the point of theoretical saturation has been reached;
- a set of categories and subcategories that represent the data that have been obtained during the study.

Elements of grounded theory

Shortly before his death, Strauss named three basic elements that should be included in every piece of research that uses the grounded theory approach (Legewie & Schervier-Legewie 2004). These are:

1. **Theoretical sensitive coding** – generating theoretical and strong concepts from the data to explain the phenomenon that is being researched.
2. **Theoretical sampling** – deciding whom to interview or what to observe next according to the state of theory generation. This means that it is essential to start data analysis with the first interview, and write down memos and hypotheses early, rather than leave it until later or even until the end of the study.
3. **The need to compare between different phenomena and contexts** – in order to make the theory strong.

Data collection

There are several data collection methods used in grounded theory, including:

- individual interviews;
- observation;
- diaries;
- focus groups.

These are discussed in chapter 8.

Note that flexibility is very important in the process of data collection for a grounded theory study because the research study, including data collection, is continually evolving as a result of the data that have already been collected. Questioning and observation will therefore be informed by the theory as it emerges. It is not a static process, but a dynamic one.

Research questions

The research question in a grounded theory study is a statement that identifies the phenomenon to be studied. The research question states what will be focused on and also what questions will be addressed. Grounded theory questions tend to be concerned with 'actions' and 'processes'.

The initial question in a grounded theory study is generally very broad, but then becomes progressively more focused as various concepts and their relationships are found to be relevant/irrelevant. This is very different from, for example, a quantitative research study where the question is refined and focused before any data are collected, and the data will either support or fail to support the question.

Advantages and disadvantages

As with all research methodologies, there are advantages and disadvantages inherent to the methodology.

Advantages
Grounded theory provides for:

- a systematic and rigorous procedure;
- rich data, which arise from the experiences of individuals who are taking part in the research study.

Disadvantages
These are:

- The subjectivity of the data leads to difficulties in establishing reliability and validity of approaches and information.
- It is difficult to detect or prevent researcher-induced bias.
- The presentation of results – the highly qualitative nature of the results can make them difficult to present in a way that practitioners can use.

Summary
- Grounded theory is an approach for looking systematically at (mostly) qualitative data and is aimed at the generation of theory from the collected data.
- Grounded theory categorises empirically collected data to build a general theory that will fit the data. (Empirical refers to information that is gained by means of observation, experience, or experiment, rather than on theory.)

Phenomenology (see also the web program)

Phenomenology comes from the academic disciplines of philosophy and psychology, and is based on the works of the twentieth-century German philosopher Edmund Husserl. It was later developed by the German philosopher Martin Heidegger.

Introduction

In its broadest sense, phenomenology refers to a person's perception of the meaning of an event, as opposed to the event as it exists externally to (outside of) that person. The focus of phenomenological inquiry is what people experience with regard to some phenomenon or other and how they interpret those experiences.

A phenomenological research study attempts to understand people's perceptions, perspectives and understandings of a particular situation or phenomenon. So we can say that phenomenology is a research method or study that tries to understand human experience by analysing a person's description of that experience. In other words, a phenomenological research study attempts to answer the question: 'What is it like to experience such and such?'

By looking at multiple perspectives of the same situation, a researcher can start to make some generalisations of what something is like as an experience from the 'insider's' perspective.

What is phenomenology?

The objective of the philosophical concept of phenomenology is the direct investigation and description of phenomena as they are consciously experienced and without the imposition of any theories that there may be about their causal explanations or their objective reality. It therefore seeks to understand how people construct meaning from their personal experiences, without reference to other people's experiences of the same phenomena.

Main characteristics of phenomenology

There are several characteristics that help to define what phenomenology is as a research methodology.

In phenomenology, the objective of the research process is the direct investigation and description of phenomena as they are consciously experienced, without theories about the causal explanations or their objective reality intruding. Therefore, within a research environment, phenomenology seeks to understand how the research participants construct meaning from their experiences of various phenomena. It investigates experiences as they are lived by those experiencing them and the meaning that these people attach to them, and bears no relation to what other people construe as their experiences.

Basically, critical truths of existence and reality are grounded in people's perceptions of their lived experiences.

There are four aspects of these lived experiences, namely:

- **Lived space** – this is difficult to define as the experience is mainly non-verbal and is not something that we normally reflect on: we simply know that the space in which we find ourselves affects how we feel. It is space as a qualitative dimension, as opposed to the physical dimension with which we are more familiar.

- **Lived body** – this is also difficult to define, but in essence is the body as a repository for our feelings. According to Brenner (2006), abstract feelings (e.g. shame, love, enjoyment) are only perceived and felt in the body. Thus, the body is an organ which, because it feels, lets feelings reach subjective reality. This is a totally different concept from the physical body and the body is seen as a living entity which is 'us'.
- **Lived time** – this bears no relation to actual time, but is our perception of time and how it influences our lives. We have all experienced periods when the minutes appear to drag (usually when we are bored) and when hours flash by (usually when we are enjoying something). In addition, there is the phenomenon that we experience of relative time – the hours and days can seem to be very long when we are children, but flash past as we get older. This is because the time that we experience is relative to our lived experiences.
- **Lived human relations** – this is perhaps the easiest of these four lived experiences to understand and implies that we live/exist through our relationships to other people.

So you can see that the four lived experiences that embody phenomenology are abstract experiences rather than physical ones, and indeed that the concept of 'being' as opposed to 'living' is an abstract constrict that we experience.

Phenomenology consists mainly of in-depth conversations, and in phenomenology, the researcher and the informants are often considered as co-participants. A very important characteristic that underlies the philosophy is that phenomenology, unlike ethnography, is person-centred rather than concerned with social processes, cultures or traditions.

Methodology
A phenomenological study often involves:

- bracketing;
- intuiting;
- analysing;
- describing.

Bracketing
Bracketing is the process of identifying and putting on hold any preconceived beliefs and opinions that one may have about the phenomenon that is being researched. The researcher 'brackets out' (as in mathematics) the world and any presuppositions that he/she may have in an effort to confront the data in as pure a form as possible. This is the central component of phenomenological reduction – the

isolation of the pure phenomenon versus what is already known of the phenomenon.

Intuiting

Intuition occurs when the researcher remains open to the meanings attributed to the phenomenon by those who have experienced it. This process results in a common understanding about the phenomenon that is being studied. Intuiting requires that the researcher creatively varies the data that are being collected until such an understanding emerges. Intuiting requires that the researcher becomes totally immersed in the study and the phenomenon.

Analysing

Analysis in phenomenological research involves coding (open, axial and selective – see chapter 9), categorising and making sense of the essential meanings of the phenomenon.

   As the researcher works and lives with the rich descriptive data that are obtained by this method, so common themes, or 'essences', begin to emerge (Essences are the ultimate structures of consciousness.) Descriptive psychology has to begin from a precise and attentive inspection of mental processes in which all assumptions about the causation, consequences and wider significance of the mental processes under inspection are eliminated.

   This stage basically involves total immersion of the researcher in the data for as long as necessary in order to ensure both a pure and a thorough description of the phenomenon.

Describing

In the descriptive stage, the researcher comes to understand and define the phenomenon. The aims of this final step are to communicate and to offer a distinct, critical description in writing and verbally. The genuine phenomenological inquiry is a matter of describing.

Sampling

Small samples (probably no more than ten participants) are most suitable for this type of research. Large samples can be unwieldy.

Data collection methods

The data collection tools that are most often used are:

- Interviews – communication through speech.
- Diaries – written communication.
- Drawings – non-verbal communication.
- Observation – visual communication.

In phenomenological philosophy and methodology with all of these data collection methods the aim is to ensure that only open questions are asked.

Advantages and disadvantages

As with all research methodologies, there are inherent advantages and disadvantages.

Advantages
Phenomenology provides for:

- an in-depth understanding of individual phenomena;
- the obtaining of rich data based on the experiences of individuals.

Disadvantages
The disadvantages are these:

- The subjectivity of the data leads to difficulties in establishing the reliability and validity of approaches and information.
- It is difficult to detect or prevent researcher-induced bias.
- There can be difficulty in ensuring pure bracketing; this can bias the interpretation of the data.
- The presentation of results – the highly qualitative nature of the results can make them difficult to present in a manner that practitioners can use.
- Phenomenology does not produce generalisable data.
- Because the samples are generally very small, can we ever say that the experiences are typical?
- The original Husserlian/Heideggerian texts were written in German, and in translation may have lost the special meaning assigned to them by the original philosophers.
- On a practical note it is important to consider the potential difficulties of participants expressing themselves.
- Participants need to be both interested and articulate. Problems that can cause difficulties in being able to express themselves include language, age, brain damage/dysfunction and embarrassment.

Conclusion

The aim of phenomenological research is to aspire to pure self-expression on the part of the participant, with non-interference from the researcher. This means there must be no 'leading questions' and the researcher completing the process of bracketing so that they can be aware of their own ideas and prejudices about the phenomenon of interest.

The phenomenological approach is especially useful when a phenomenon of interest has been poorly defined or conceptualised – or you did not even know it existed!

According to Van Manen (1990), the four aspects of 'lived experience' that are of interest to phenomenologists are:

- lived space (the concept of spatiality);
- lived body (the concept of corporeality);

- lived time (the concept of temporality);
- lived human relations (the concept of relationality).

The topics appropriate to phenomenological research studious are those that are fundamental to the life experiences of humans, such as:

- the meaning of health/stress;
- the experience of bereavement;
- the quality of life with a chronic illness.

Phenomenology may encompass narrative research. Narrative research is a story of the day/week/year/life in the lives of individuals as told by these individuals. The researcher re-tells or 're-stories' this into a narrative chronology, combining views taken from the participants' and the researcher's lives. Phenomenology is attractive to qualitative nurse researchers because caring (Heidegger uses the German word 'Sorge') is fundamental to the research approach. Phenomenology can be a vehicle to illuminate and clarify central issues in nursing.

All this may seems very philosophical and possibly a little complex, but put simply, phenomenology is the understanding of personal truth, in which the only truth that exists for an individual is what that individual perceives to be true, so within one house, let alone the world, there can be as many 'truths' of an experience/phenomenon as there are people living there, and the role of the phenomenological researcher is to try to get them to explain their version of the 'truth' and make sense of it, and then compare it with the 'truths' of others undergoing the same experience/phenomenon.

Data collection methods

Finally, in qualitative research, there are many data collection methods that can be used to collect data, including:

- individual interviews;
- focus groups;
- observation;
- diaries;
- drawings.

These are discussed in chapter 8.

Qualitative research: summary

'Qualitative research is a systematic, subjective approach used to describe life experiences and give them meaning' (Burns & Grove 2005: 52).

Qualitative research allows us to gain insights into phenomena associated with people and their lives. But, more importantly, it allows us to try to find meanings to phenomena and events experienced by people, and to their life experiences in general.

As Burns & Grove (2005) point out, the insights that we gain as qualitative researchers are not necessarily linked to, and understood through, the causes of the phenomena and other experiences, but rather through an understanding of the 'whole' experiences of the participants in our studies. Therefore, we work within a holistic framework, and this allows us to explore the depth, richness and complexity that are inherent in phenomena that are experienced by others and ourselves.

Summary

This chapter has explored the various elements that you have to consider when designing a research study. Most importantly, you will need to ensure that:

- you have a research question/hypothesis that will allow you to research exactly what you are interested in;
- your research design is the most appropriate one for the problem that you are investigating.

Once these two conditions have been met, the rest of your research proposal (and your research) will flow naturally because the basics are right.

Activity

Take a topic in which you are interested (this need not be work-related) and write a research question or hypothesis on one aspect only of that topic.

- How will you decide whether you are going to write a research question or a hypothesis?
- Now decide which paradigm would best explore your research question/ hypothesis.
- Make a list of all the pros and cons of using your chosen paradigm to explore your research question/hypothesis.

References

Brenner A. (2006) The lived body and the dignity of human being. In H. L. Dreyfus & M. A. Wrathall (Eds.) *A Companion to phenomenology and existentialism* (pp. 478–488). Chichester: Wiley-Blackwell.

Bunkers S. S., Petardi L. A., Pilkington F.B. & Walls P. A. (1996) Challenging the myths surrounding qualitative research in nursing. *Nursing Science Quarterly* **9**: 33–37.

Burns N. & Grove S. K. (2005) *The practice of nursing research: conduct, critique, and utilization* (5th edition). St. Louis, MO: Elsevier Saunders.

Creswell J. W. (1994) *Research design: Qualitative and quantitative approaches.* London: Sage.

Crookes P. A. & Davies S. (2004) *Research into practice: Essential skills for reading and applying research in nursing and health care* (2nd edition). Edinburgh: Baillière Tindall.

Flanagan J. C. (1954) The critical incident technique. *Psychological Bulletin* **51**(4): 327–359.

Glaser B. G. & Strauss A. L. (1967) *The discovery of grounded theory. Strategies for qualitative research.* Chicago: Aldine Publishing Co.

Hammersley M. (1992) The generalisability of ethnography. In M. Hammersley, *What's wrong with ethnography?* (pp. 85–95). London: Routledge.

Holloway I. (2005) *Qualitative research in health care.* London: Sage.

Jasper M. (2003) *Beginning reflective practice.* Cheltenham: Nelson Thorne.

Leedy P. D. & Ormrod J. E. (2005) *Practical research: Planning and design* (8th edition). Englewood Cliffs, NJ: Pearson Merrill Prentice Hall.

Legewie H. & Schervier-Legewie B. (2004) Forschung ist harte Arbeit, es ist immer ein Stück Leiden damit verbunden. Deshalb muss es auf der anderen Seite Spaß machen. *Forum: Qualitative Social Research On-line Journal*, **5**(3): Art. 22.

Norbeck J. S. (1987) In defence of empiricism. *Image – Journal of Nursing Scholarship* **19**(1): 28–30.

Parahoo K. (1997) *Nursing research: Principles, process and issues.* Basingstoke: Macmillan.

Peat J., Mellis C., Williams K. and Xuan W. (2002) *Health Science Research: A handbook of quantitative methods.* London: Sage.

Polit D. F. & Hungler B. P. (1999) *Nursing research: Principles and methods* (6th edition). Philadelphia: Lippincott.

Porter S. & Carter D. E. (2000) Common terms and concepts in research. In D. Cormack (Ed.) *The Research process in nursing* (4th edition) (pp. 17–28). Oxford: Blackwell Science.

Van Manen M. (1990) *Researching lived experience: Human science for an action sensitive pedagogy.* London, Ontario: Althouse.

Weaver K. & Olson J. K. (2006) Understanding paradigms used for nursing research. *Journal of Advanced Nursing* **53**(4): 459–469.

Scenario – Possible suggestions

You may have come up with two possible types of research that you could use for your study. These are:

- descriptive research;
- survey research.

Descriptive research may be your choice because you will be describing what exists, and what you describe could be used as a springboard for further investigations into this phenomenon: Is it linked to environmental factors, or employment factors? Are there clusters, or is the phenomenon evenly spread? Is gender a factor?

However, you may choose survey research, because that is what it is that you will be performing – a survey.

The Research Proposal: Ethics in Research

Introduction

This chapter is linked to the ethics section of the web program. When preparing for a research study, ethical approval is essential. You have already learned that, when carrying out an investigation, the researcher must have the knowledge and expertise to be able to undertake it, but of equal importance is that the work must be conducted in a manner that requires honesty and integrity. Such transparency must be evident throughout the entire research process, starting with the selection of the research topic, through to the presentation and publication of the study findings. However, underpinning everything is that all research must be carried out ethically, and much of the preparation of your research proposal and the actual research is concerned with ensuring that your proposed research will be ethical in all its aspects. This chapter introduces you to the concept, role and practicalities of ethics in research and shows you how you can prepare the ethical component of your research proposal.

Introduction to ethics

Ethics is a branch of philosophy and refers to moral values and moral conduct (Singer 1993, Porter 2000). It is also a method, procedure or view for deciding how to act when analysing complex issues (Porter 2000, Parahoo 2006). Put simply, ethical behaviour refers to what is 'in accordance with principles of conduct that are considered correct, especially those of a given profession or group' (Collins Dictionary 1986: 289). In this chapter we are concerned with the principles of conduct relating to health research. The chapter also addresses some of the issues pertaining to ethics committees. The discussion of ethics in this chapter is given in the context of current healthcare research policy in the UK by exploring key components of research governance and research and development (R&D) approval. The chapter concludes by looking at points to bear in mind when critiquing the ethics of research studies.

But first, it is important to note that ethics and research have not always gone hand in hand and, in the past, some historical and current ethical transgressions have taken place in a number of notable studies, which have led to the establishment of a code of conduct to which all researchers must adhere. Before considering how you can ensure that your research is ethically sound, we shall look at some of these transgressions so you can see how far we have come in the last few years in terms of ethical research.

Ethical transgressions in research

The Nazi medical experiments 1933–45: Experiments were conducted on prisoners of war and people in concentration camps, without their consent, to investigate:

- endurance (e.g. exposure to high altitudes, freezing temperatures);
- untested drug tolerance, poisons;
- malaria;
- torture;
- typhus;
- surgical procedures, usually performed without anaesthesia (Belmont Report 1979).

An examination of the Nazis' records shows that the research was poorly conceived and conducted, and yielded questionable benefits – as well as being often fatal to the victims of the research, with the vast majority dying during or just after the procedure (Belmont Report, 1979).

The second example of ethical violations in research concerns the Tuskegee syphilis study that took place between 1932 and 1972 in the United States. This Public Health Service-initiated study investigated 400 African-American men in Alabama in order to determine the natural course of syphilis. Medical treatment for the disease was withheld from the men for the purpose of the research study. Participants were not informed of the reason and procedures of the research and so could not give their consent, informed or otherwise (Belmont Report 1979).

Third is the Jewish Chronic Disease Hospital study of 1963. This study was conducted in order to look at patients' rejection of live cancer cells. As with the Tuskegee syphilis study, patients were not informed that they were in a research study and so did not give their consent, nor were they told that they were being injected with live cancer cells. Crucially, the study did not have ethics approval, even though the researchers knew that it was required (Belmont Report 1979).

Not all the problems with unethical research are to be found in the past. More recently, inquiries have been conducted into the removal of organs and tissues from deceased patients without the consent of their relatives (Bristol Royal Infirmary Report 2001, Royal Liverpool Children's Inquiry Report 2001). These inquiries called into question the conduct of some of the health professionals concerned.

These conflicts in research have given rise to a code of ethics or a guide/framework all healthcare professionals have to adhere to, and which helps researchers ensure that their research is ethical and is put in place in order to protect participants and researchers alike.

Code of ethics

The first internationally recognised code was the Nuremberg Code of 1949 which emanated from the Nuremberg Trials of Nazi war criminals which were held after the Second World War when the researchers involved in the Nazi experiments were brought to trial. The Code includes guidance regarding:

- the consent process;
- the protection of participants from harm;
- taking into account the balance of risks and benefits inherent in a study

(Fry & Johnstone 2008).

The Nuremberg Code laid the foundation for the Helsinki Declaration (1964, as revised and updated in the 1970s, 1980s, 1990s and most recently in 2008). Three of the key principles of the Helsinki Declaration suggest that:

- the researchers should have respect for the individual's right to self-determination and to make informed decisions regarding participating in the research;
- the participants' welfare should override the interests of science and society;
- special attention should be given to vulnerable individuals and groups

(World Medical Association 2008).

In addition to these international codes, most disciplines have their own code of ethics. For example, the UK's Nursing and Midwifery Council (2004), the Royal College of Nursing (2007) and The Chartered Society of Physiotherapy (2001) have all published standards for performance for their professionals. Areas covered in these codes include:

- informed consent;
- confidentiality;
- data protection;

- the right to withdraw from the study;
- any potential benefits and harm;
- the maintenance of professional knowledge and competence.

These values are shared by all UK healthcare professionals (Nursing and Midwifery Council 2004) and have to be evident in your research proposal, and of course in the research study itself.

Thus, all research should be undertaken in accordance with widely agreed principles such as those laid down in the Helsinki Declaration.

Having discussed the background to why we have to include ethical dimensions in all our research, we can turn to what these ethical principles are and how we apply them.

Ethical principles

Ethical principles can be found in the web program, in particular Beauchamp & Childress's (2001) four principles which we are going to discuss next. The four principles approach is an internationally used framework which aims to address ethical issues. The four principles are:

- respect for autonomy;
- beneficence;
- non-maleficence;
- justice.

Although we are concentrating on these four, it is important to acknowledge, as some authors do (e.g. Beauchamp & Childress 2001, Storch et al. 2004, Parahoo 2006), that there are three more principles to cover in our research proposal and research study, namely:

- fidelity;
- veracity;
- confidentiality.

So our discussion will cover all seven.

Respect for autonomy (see the web program)
Respect for autonomy obliges the researcher to respect the participant's informed decision whether or not to participate in the research study. This means that the researcher must ensure that the participant has full information about what the study entails, including any risks and benefits, and is given sufficient time to reflect on the information and to ask any questions they may have about the research and their role in it. This ensures that they enter into the research study voluntarily and with all the information that they need to make an informed decision as to whether or not to take part. Another aspect of respect for autonomy that we, as researchers, have to ensure occurs is that no

participants are coerced, however important the study may be. In addition, the participants should be told that they have the right to withdraw at any stage without adverse consequences to them.

Another essential responsibility for the researcher preparing a research proposal is that there are mechanisms in place for ensuring that the confidentiality of the participants is fully maintained. This is crucial in any research study, and ethics committees scrutinise this aspect of the research proposal very carefully (see below).

Gelling (1999) proposes three types of autonomy:

1. **Autonomy of thought** – this includes a wide range of intellectual activities described as 'thinking for oneself'.
2. **Autonomy of will** – this involves the freedom of the individual to do something based on their own deliberations.
3. **Autonomy of action** – this states that once the decision has been made, the individual should be able to act as she/he wishes.

Thus you can see that the right to self-determination and to be fully informed are key elements on which informed consent is based (Polit & Beck 2004).

Now we come to be thorny part of ethics and research: some groups are deemed to have diminished levels of autonomy or self-determination (e.g. those with cognitive impairment, the terminally ill, young children) or situations that severely restrict their liberty (e.g. prisoners or people compulsorily detained under the Mental Health Act), and it is absolutely crucial that such individuals are given additional protection to ensure that the principle of respect for autonomy is upheld (this issue is discussed later in the chapter).

Beneficence (see the web program)
The principle of beneficence requires the researcher to act in the best interests of the participant, according to their professional assessment. It requires the researcher 'to do good' with his/her research, so this has to be planned into the research proposal and the research study itself, and then a system of monitoring has to be installed in the research protocol. Monitoring the research ensures that it is being undertaken as envisaged during the planning phase (and must be included in the research proposal). Silverman (2007) points out that monitoring involves the researcher (and anyone connected with the research) sticking rigidly to approved protocols, including the full documentation of any adverse events (particularly in clinical trials) and ensuring the integrity of the data collected.

Thus, beneficence can be seen to be the most important principle for nurses and other health professionals involved in clinical research to be aware of and to act on, because it concerns the protection of patients by ensuring that the central tenet of 'do no harm' remains at the forefront of the research study.

But how can we determine that our research really is beneficial – that is, how can we be certain that the principle of beneficence applies to our research study? This is something for you to think about. One of the ways in which you can try to ensure beneficence is by adhering to ethical principles as you write and think about your research proposal and your study. Obtaining help and guidance from more senior researchers will also help you to make sure that you have applied the principle of beneficence. Another suggestion is to try to put yourself in the place of the participants and ask yourself questions such as: Would I like that procedure to be done to me or would I like to be asked that question? Fortunately, there is enough guidance in current practice and from our earlier training to ensure that we do not stray too far from the principle of beneficence in our dealings with patients and clients. However, it is worthwhile pointing out that the principle of benefi-cence is not always as straightforward as it may appear to be. Gener-ally, as healthcare professionals we are concerned with alleviating suffering and saving lives, but sometimes we can be faced with a dilemma. For example, Dubois (2005) argues that in palliative medicine stopping treatment, in an appropriate clinical context, may be viewed as an act of beneficence when the continuation of life is viewed by the patient as harmful. Examples like this are what make ethics such an interesting, but at times frustrating, subject.

However, much of the principle of beneficence is quite clear-cut – all you have to do is ask yourself: 'Will this be of benefit to the patient/client?'

Examples of beneficence include:

- providing vaccinations for the general population;
- encouraging a patient to stop smoking;
- starting an exercise programme and encouraging healthy eating in particular groups.

Now let's look at these examples in more detail. Are they always beneficent? That depends on your viewpoint and this is where bias in its broadest sense comes into play. If you believe in the efficacy of vac-cinations in preventing ill-health, then you would certainly say that the first example is beneficial. However, the parents of a child who, after receiving the MMR vaccination, is found to be autistic may have a dif-ferent view. Whether the MMR vaccination has actually caused the child's autism is immaterial – it is the parents' perception that matters to them in deciding whether the vaccination adheres to the principle of beneficence.

Turn now to the second example. Is stopping smoking always ben-eficial? Well, as healthcare professionals, we would say yes every time. It is certainly better for physical health, but what about psychological well-being? Suppose that you perceive that the only enjoyable thing in your life is smoking – would you agree that giving up smoking is beneficial to you? And what about someone who is dying and enjoys a cigarette – is the risk of their contracting cardiovascular disease or lung cancer still a worry? Again, it is the individual who is important here. The same argument applies to the third example.

What we hope that you have come to realise is that nothing is carved in stone – we have to look at individual cases (something we are taught to do as healthcare professionals), and we should take the same stance with potential participants and subjects in our proposed research studies. This is why we said that, as you are planning your research study and starting to write your research proposal, you should try to put yourself in the place of the potential participants and subjects of your study, and ask yourself: 'What in this study is beneficial to me and what is not?'

Non-maleficence (see the web program)
The third of our ethical principles – non-maleficence – complements beneficence and assumes that intentional harm to participants is prevented. In current clinical care, many beneficial therapies also have associated risks – think of the potential adverse reactions listed in the information that accompanies medicines and you will see the truth in this statement.

Consequently, we have to accept that there is the potential for harm in even the ethically best designed research study, So, when preparing our research proposal, we have to accept this and try to minimise any risks (and also have some means of countering any adverse reactions, whether these are physical, emotional or psychosocial) that may occur during our research study. We also have to look at the key ethical consideration in all research, namely, do the benefits outweigh the risks?

Research should benefit the participant by contributing to their welfare and/or that of society as a whole (Parahoo 2006).This is discussed at length in the context of palliative care in the web program (see under ethics there).

Thus the concepts of weighing the potential benefit to the patient against the potential harm, along with the patient's stated views, are employed in healthcare decision-making. Consider again a dying patient (an area of great controversy in healthcare) and continuing aggressive, life-prolonging treatment can be seen as a violation of non-maleficence (Dubois 2005). Similarly, euthanasia, along with the premature, unrequested or uninformed withdrawal of treatment, may also be viewed as violations of non-maleficence (Dubois 2005).

Justice (see the web program)
The fourth ethical principle – justice – requires the researcher to be fair to participants by acting impartially. Of great importance in the use of this principle is that the needs of the participants should come before

the objectives of the study; similarly, vulnerable groups should not be used merely for the researcher's convenience (Parahoo 2006). Polit & Beck (2004) explain that fair treatment means that:

- The selection of participants must be based on research requirements and not on the vulnerability or compromised position of the individual.
- Participants have the right to fair and equitable treatment before, during and after participating in the study.
- The researcher is obliged to honour all promises and commitments made in the research proposal.
- Courtesy and tact are expected at all times.
- Participants have the right to non-prejudicial treatment if they decide to withdraw from the study.
- Participants should have access to feedback to clarify issues raised in the study.
- Participants should have access to professional help in the event of physical and/or psychological damage as a result of the study.
- Researchers should show respect for different cultural beliefs.

In essence, the principle of justice is seen in the research process by there being a fair and equitable distribution of benefits and burdens, as well as fairness in the selection of research subjects (Khan et al. 1998, Aita & Richer 2005).

Having looked briefly at the four basic ethical principles, we now turn our attention to the other three principles as identified by Beauchamp & Childress (2001), Parahoo (2006) and Storch et al. (2004), namely fidelity, veracity and confidentiality.

Fidelity

Fidelity refers to the building of trust between the participant/subject and the researcher (ICN 2006). Research participants entrust themselves to the researcher, who has an obligation to safeguard their welfare. They should be told of the risks of the study when the researcher is seeking their consent. This is very closely linked to beneficence and non-maleficence, and is just as important because the researcher and the participant/subject in effect make a contract, which is formalised by the signing and witnessing of the consent form.

Veracity

This principle is linked to the basic principles of respect for autonomy, beneficence and non-maleficence and it obliges the researcher to be truthful about the study, even if in so doing potential participants are deterred from entering the study (Polit & Beck 2008). Although linked to these three basic principles, veracity is more closely linked to the principle of autonomy (Gillon 1994). Patients' autonomy is infringed if information that may contribute to their informed decision-making is withheld from them. Consequently, if their autonomy is infringed or not heeded, they are not able to make a fully informed decision.

Confidentiality

The issue of confidentiality is discussed in the web program under ethics. Ensuring the confidentiality and privacy of research data is a key principle in the research process and is very closely scrutinised by the research ethics committee. In order to reduce the risk of identifying the participants from their comments or other data, many researchers use identification numbers or pseudonyms so that only the researchers and the participants can make the connection between comments and other data and their identity. Protecting identity and confidentiality extends to the dissemination of findings (see chapter 10 and the web program). Another important consideration, particularly when writing up and disseminating your findings, is that you should make sure that the research site(s) as well as the participants cannot be identified, because it may be possible to identify the participants (patients/clients or other healthcare professionals) if the research site(s) are known.

Summary

This has been a brief look at the principles that underlie any ethical research study; it is important to be aware of them and to be comfortable with them because they are the principles that guide our ethical and professional conduct when we are involved in any research. We acknowledge that although we have given you information on, and have stressed the importance of, these principles, the fact remains that they cannot cover all eventualities that you may come across as a researcher. Therefore, we have to stress, as indeed all responsible organisations do, that as registered professionals we must take responsibility for all our actions no matter the situation or environment in which we work, whether we are acting as clinical practitioners or as researchers.

You will find more on this subject in the accompanying web program.

Research ethics committees

Now we turn to research ethics committees. Unfortunately, the words 'research ethics committee' produce an anxious state in some researchers. This is often the result of having previously submitted a research proposal that was rejected. This is unfortunate because our experience has been overwhelmingly positive, and we have found them to be generally very helpful, caring, insightful and, above all, friendly.

Some countries have a single system to which applicants can apply for approval to undertake research, but if you do not live in the UK you should discuss the system in your country with an experienced researcher. In the UK, the Integrated Research Application System (IRAS) is the dataset we use as the instrument for applying for permissions and approvals for health and social care/community care research. It is an integrated research application system which captures the information needed to submit for approval. It replaces duplication of applications and helps to meet the regulatory and governance requirements of research projects. (For more information on this, go to www.rdforum.nhs.uk/docs/irasbrochure.pdf.) In addition, the web program has a direct link to the Integrated Research Application Process (www.myresearchproject.org.uk) and here you can access the research ethics form, as well as information on completing it.

Information you have to supply

The research ethics form contains many questions, from the straight-forward (e.g. name of research project, your personal details), to those about the proposed research, and in particular its ethics. Below is a sample of the questions that you have to answer, just to give you a flavour of them. You will see that for many there are instructions as to what is required, so filling in the form is simple – as long as you have written a good research proposal!

Sample of questions from IRAS form

A6-1. Summary of the study. *Please provide a brief summary of the research (maximum 300 words) using language easily understood by lay reviewers and members of the public. This summary will be published on the website of the National Research Ethics Service following the ethical review.*

A6-2. Summary of main issues. *Please summarise the main ethical and design issues arising from the study and say how you have addressed them.*

A10. What is the principal research question/objective? *Please put this in language comprehensible to a lay person.*

A13. Please give a full summary of your design and methodology. *It should be clear exactly what will happen to the research participant, how many times and in what order. Please complete this section in language comprehensible to the lay person. Do not simply reproduce or refer to the protocol. Further guidance is available in the guidance notes.*

A14-1. In which aspects of the research process have you actively involved, or will you involve, patients, service users or members of the public?

A22. What are the potential risks and burdens for research participants and how will you minimise then? *For all studies, describe any potential adverse effects, pain, discomfort, distress, intrusion, inconvenience or changes to lifestyle. Only describe risks or burdens that could occur as a result of participation in the research. Say what steps would be taken to minimise risks and burdens as far as possible.*

A23. Will interviews/questionnaires or group discussions include topics that might be sensitive, embarrassing or upsetting, or is it possible that criminal or other disclosures requiring action could occur during the study?

A30-1. Will you obtain informed consent from or on behalf of research participants?

☑ Yes ☐ No

If you will be obtaining consent from adult participants, please give details of who will take consent and how it will be done, with details of any steps to provide information (a written information sheet, videos, or interactive material). Arrangements for adults unable to consent for themselves should be described separately in Part B Section 6, and for children in Part B Section 7.

If you plan to seek informed consent from vulnerable groups, say how you will ensure that consent is voluntary and fully informed.

A38. How will you ensure the confidentiality of personal data?
Please provide a general statement of the policy and procedures for ensuring confidentiality, e.g. anonymisation or pseudonymisation of data.

A43. How long will personal data be stored or accessed after the study has ended?

A51. How do you intend to report and disseminate the results of the study?

A59. What is the sample size for the research? *How many participants/samples/ data records do you plan to study in total? If there is more than one group, please give further details below.*

A62. Please describe the methods of analysis (statistical or other appropriate methods, e.g. for qualitative research) by which the data will be evaluated to meet the study objectives.

(IRAS 2008)

A checklist is also provided specifying which documents you have to submit, along with this form. As was pointed out above, filling in the IRAS form is quite simple as long as you have written your research proposal well because many of the questions can be answered by simply cutting and pasting them from the research proposal. At the same time, this form can help you to formulate your research proposal because it acts as a checklist you can refer to in order to ensure that your research proposal includes all the relevant information.

With this system you will find that the process of organising and going through the ethics approval procedure has been much simplified over recent years, particularly if you wish to undertake your research at several sites (known as multi-site research), such as hospitals and clinics. In the past, each one of these sites would have had its own research ethics committee and each its own forms to fill in and procedures to go through. This was both stressful and very time-consuming. So, you will be pleased to hear that now you apply to just one research committee and, if your research is approved, it is automatically approved for all sites in the UK.

The only exception arises when you are undertaking research that is particularly sensitive, there are other concerns (e.g. research with vulnerable people) or there is a greater than normal potential risk involved. In these cases, although the ethics research committee may give their approval, it is subject to what is known as 'Site Specific Assessment'. This means that each of the sites in which you wish to undertake your research must give their approval. Again, this is not as great a problem as it used to be because they will accept the form that you have used for the main research ethics committee if it includes a brief addendum which is specific to that site.

Site-Specific Assessment

One of the authors undertook research which included interviewing patients undergoing palliative care about their experiences. This is a sensitive topic and many of the interviewees were very vulnerable because they were terminally ill (some died during the course of the research study). For these reasons, as well as the fact that the research was undertaken at four sites, before ethics approval could be granted, each of the sites had to give their approval after the main committee had done so. There was no need for the researcher to meet the committees, and all were happy to approve the research, which was subsequently successfully completed.

So who sits on these research ethics committees which can produce such a range of emotions in researchers? A research ethics committee is a group of independent people made up of health professionals and members of the public, including service users and carers, whose main functions are to ensure objectively the protection of research participants by reviewing, approving and monitoring the research study. This multidisciplinary approach can provide diverse viewpoints on ethical issues because each member brings their own experience, viewpoints and biases. Before you, as a researcher, meet them, they will have received your research ethics form (see below) and had the opportunity to read it and think about it. Then they will have discussed it together as a research ethics committee before holding their meeting with you. When they do meet you, they will have agreed the points they wish to discuss with you and the recommendations/suggestions that they may want to make. Your role as a researcher is to discuss your proposed research with them and demonstrate its value and ethical soundness. The members of the research ethics committee may then seek clarification on specific points before making a recommendation (National Patient Safety Agency 2007).

Vulnerability in research

At this point, it is useful to discuss briefly vulnerability and research, because this has been mentioned several times in this chapter and comprises an important part of the IRAS form.

The *Shorter Oxford English Dictionary* (2007) defines vulnerable as being 'able to be wounded, able to be physically or emotionally hurt, liable to damage or harm'. From that, you can see that any participant in a drugs trial, such as one that involves a change of treatment, is vulnerable because they are at risk of being physically harmed. However, there is another type of vulnerable participant in a research study, and that is anybody who is at risk of emotional harm.

Children are classed as vulnerable because they may not be aware of, or understand, what they are being asked to do when taking part in a research study whether it is quantitative or qualitative in design. In addition, they may not be emotionally mature enough to cope with the study. There is the problem of them being able to give informed consent. Other classes of vulnerable research participants are patients with special needs, those with mental health problems, those who are seriously ill, those who are dying and foetuses.

However, a case can be made for treating everybody who takes part in the research as vulnerable. Patients/clients are vulnerable for the very reason that they are sick or have other problems. At the same time, non-patients/clients who take part in research, such as you as a healthcare professional, can be considered to be vulnerable if you are participating in research because, like patients and clients, during the research study you are letting someone else (i.e. the researcher) into your life, and this can make you feel and be vulnerable.

The simple solution is to treat everybody who is taking part in research as vulnerable, even though some may be more vulnerable than others. The important thing is not to pre-judge the vulnerability of participants and subjects in a research study, but to try to put in place safeguards to protect them. In particular, during your contact with participants be on your guard and look out for signs of vulnerability and distress (do not exclude yourself from the risk of vulnerability and distress). For example, one of the authors who undertook research into palliative care found the interviews with the patients and their families emotionally very draining and had to rethink the approach to the interviews and find someone who could lend support.

The question now is this: How do we offset the risk of harm (physical, psychosocial, emotional) to the participants and the researcher?

1. It is important that you make provisions for support before the research study starts, rather than part way through when damage may have been done, and it may not be so easy to arrange such support.
2. Ensure that you have given the potential participants all the information that will help them make an informed decision as to whether or not to take

part in the research study. You have to look at ways of communicating this information, particularly to children and those with special needs.

3. You must be responsive not only to what the participants say during the research study, but to their non-verbal cues as well.

4. Finally, be prepared to stop an interview, or drugs trial, if you feel that the participants or subjects are becoming distressed or are suffering any sort of harm.

You will see examples of how researchers can attempt to minimise risk of harm when you work through the two research proposal examples in the ethics section of the web program.

Information sheets

Rather than discuss what needs to be included in an information sheet (these differ from research study to research study and from participant to participant) it is much easier for you to understand by giving you an example of an information sheet (below) for adult patients. Read it, then think what you might want to change in it from your own experience.

The effectiveness of palliative care services in .... in meeting the needs of patients with cancer and the needs of their families

You are being invited to take part in a research study. Before you decide whether or not to take part in this study, it is important for you to understand why the research is being done and what it will involve. Please take time to read the following information carefully and discuss it with others if you wish. Do contact me if there is anything that is not clear or if you would like more information. It is important that you take time to decide whether or not you wish to take part.

Thank you for reading this.

What is the purpose of the study?

Members of the palliative care team in .... are constantly striving to improve the service and care that they give in order to improve the quality of life of the people they care for. Consequently, the aims of this study are first to find out from patients with cancer, and their families and carers, what their needs are, and whether the palliative services team is meeting those needs. Secondly, this study aims to allow the patients and their families and carers to discuss how the care that they are given by the palliative care team could be improved.

Why have I been chosen?

You, along with up to 14 other patients and families/carers, were randomly chosen from all who are using palliative care services.

Do I have to take part?

No, you do not have to take part in this study; it is entirely up to you to decide whether or not take part. Whether or not you decide to take part, you will be given this information sheet to keep.

   If, after careful consideration, you do decide to take part, you will be asked to sign a consent form and return it to me in the stamped and addressed envelope attached to the consent form. You will be then sent a copy of your signed consent form to keep with this information sheet. Even if you do decide to take part and return the consent form, you are still free to withdraw from the study at any time and you do not need to give a reason. Please be assured that the decision not to take part or a decision to withdraw from the study at any time during the research will not affect the standard of care that you receive from the palliative care team.

What will happen to me if I take part?

If you do decide to take part, I, or one of my research team, will contact you to arrange a day and time that suit you in order for one of us to come to talk with you. We will be happy to meet with you in your own home or, if you would prefer, somewhere else. If you would prefer that we meet outside of your home, we will pay your travel expenses. The meeting will last between 30 and 45 minutes, and we will ask you to talk about your experiences of living with cancer and your needs regarding the care that you can obtain from the palliative care team. With your permission, we would like to tape-record our conversation. This is because we can then make notes from our conversation afterwards. This will help us to analyse everybody's thoughts, needs and suggestions, so that we can then produce a report. I would like to emphasise again that you can withdraw from the research study at any time, even during our meeting and conversation.

What are at the possible disadvantages and risks of taking part?

It is possible that, during our conversation, you may become distressed. If that were to happen, then if you wish we will not continue and the tape recorder will be switched off. If, during or following our meeting, you feel that you would like to talk to someone else about how you are feeling, you will be given details of someone whom you can contact.

What are the possible benefits of taking part?

You, along with other people taking part in this research study, will have an opportunity of informing members of the palliative care team about your needs and whether you think your needs are being met. This will allow the palliative care team to evaluate the effectiveness of their services, and, if possible, to improve them.

Will my taking part in this study be kept confidential?

Although, with your permission, the conversation will be recorded, only members of the research team will have access to the tape recording and transcripts of your recording. These will be kept in a locked cabinet at the University of .... and will be destroyed at the end of the research study, once the report has been written. No member of the palliative care team, or anyone involved in your care, will be able to identify who has or has not taken part in the research from the final report. Your own names will not be used and no personal information about yourself will be given in the final report.

What will happen to the results of the research study?

The results of the research study will be collected together and a report written. As mentioned in the paragraph above, you will not be identified in this report. This report will be sent to the palliative care team, the two primary care trusts involved in this study, the .... Hospital, and the .... Hospice. All patients and families/carers who take part in the research will be sent a copy of the results.

Results from the research will be published in professional medical and nursing journals, and will also be presented at professional conferences, in order that people from outside of .... will be able to learn from the results.

Who is organising and funding the research?

The research has been organised by a group comprising representatives from the palliative care services team and the University .... However, the actual research is organised and run only by researchers from University ....Funding for the research has come from the .... PCT (Primary Care Trust), but be assured that the researchers are independent from the .... PCT.

Who has reviewed the study?

This research study has been reviewed by the .... Research Ethics Committee and the Research Governance Committees of .... PCT, ... PCT, the .... Hospital, and the .... Hospice.

Contact for further information

If you have any further questions or wish further information, then please contact the chief researcher:..........................(name of chief researcher)

I would like to take this opportunity to thank you for taking the time to read this information sheet and, whether or not you decide to take part in the research, to thank you for considering it.

Another way of reducing the risk of emotional distress is to ensure that every communication with the participants is friendly, informative and takes account of their needs. For example, when trying to recruit participants for your research study, we find that it is very useful to have a contact sheet, so whoever makes the first contact knows how to approach it. Below is a copy of the first contact sheet for the palliative care research study.

Contact sheet – first contact by nurses

- Take with you:
  1. Summary of research study
  2. Information sheet
  3. Consent form
  4. Stamped and addressed envelope
- Explain the research to the patient/family member/carer (use summary sheet)
- Stress:
  1. They are under no obligation to take part
  2. Their care will not be affected if they do not take part
  3. Nobody in palliative care services will know who has taken part or refused – only the researchers will know
  4. The research and final report will maintain complete anonymity
  5. That they should read the information sheet carefully
  6. That they can discuss it with anyone if it helps them to make a decision
  7. If they want to take part, they sign and return the consent form in the envelope within two weeks
  8. They can contact .... (Lead Researcher) if they have any further questions or want more information
  9. They can keep the information sheet, whether or not they decide to take part in the research study
- Do allow them to ask any questions of you and answer them truthfully. Remember you probably know them better than anyone else in the palliative care team and they trust you
- Do not pressure them one way or another
- If you do not know the answer to any of their questions, tell them that you will contact the research team and get back to them.

Even with all these safeguards in place, we cannot assure you that you will have no problems with the vulnerability of your participants, but the risk will be greatly reduced.

Decisions by the research ethics committee

Following this discussion of vulnerability and how you can approach vulnerable participants, we can return to the submission of your form to the research ethics committee.

After your meeting with the committee, they can make one of five decisions on your research proposal:

1. Favourable – go ahead and get started on the research study.
2. Provisional favourable opinion subject to a Site Specific Assessment – this means that you can go ahead with your research once you have had it assessed by the potential research sites (see above).
3. Provisional opinion with a request for further information – often, these are only minor matters or concerns, and approval is often delegated to the chair of the committee on the information being satisfactorily forthcoming from the researcher.
4. No opinion – this occurs when the research ethics committee cannot decide whether to grant approval or not and wish to consult a 'specialist referee', who may be able to clarify matters so that they can then reach a decision (either favourable or unfavourable).
5. Unfavourable opinion – this is the one that all researchers want to avoid, because it means that the research ethics committee does not believe that the research application is presented well. However disappointing, it is not the end of the world because the researcher can submit their research application again:
    –   either by addressing the concerns of the research ethics committee and re-submitting the application to the committee at a later date;
    –   or by sending the same ethics research application forms to another research ethics committee following the submission of notice of appeal to the National Research Ethics Service.

(Davies 2008)

In making their decision, the ethics committee has to address various issues, including:

*   the potential risks and benefits to participants/subjects;
*   how the research study will add to our present knowledge of the topic;
*   how the potential participants/subjects will be selected (sampling);
*   if and how consent will be obtained;
*   procedures to protect the privacy and anonymity of the participants;
*   the potential involvement of vulnerable groups and how you will deal with this;
*   how, and by whom, the research study will be monitored.

In addition, the research ethics committees will require information from you. This may include:

- copies of participant information sheets;
- copies of letters to the participants;
- copies of consent forms;
- signed agreement of indemnity (if necessary);
- copies of any questionnaires/interview schedules (i.e. your data collection instruments);
- financial statements – who is sponsoring the research study.

All these are covered in the guidelines for the IRAS ethics form, which also gives information on what to submit and how to submit it.

Scenario

Depending on your role, you want to undertake research into:

- how children perceive having an x-ray;
- the importance of exercise and diet in the elderly to reduce strain on the hips;
- the risks of living rough as perceived by homeless young males;
- the importance of the father to the mother and child in the special care baby unit – a comparative study between paternal attendance and non-attendance;
- the perceptions of elderly female patients of being cared for by male nurses.

From what you have learned so far in this book and the accompanying web program, you should plan a simple research study to tackle one of these scenarios, and then compose an information sheet to let the potential participants know about the proposed study. Use the example to help you. You should pay particular attention to the possibility of vulnerability and risk to the participants – try to allay their fears and doubts.

Finally, note that, in the examples above, all the participants, for one reason or another, could be considered to be highly vulnerable. So, when designing your information sheet, you will need to take certain factors into account, including:

- their likely attention span (the elderly and children);
- their potential fear of hospitals and of hospital procedures (the elderly and children);

- their mental capacity – either because of developmental stage, old age, drug use or extreme anxiety (all of the above);
- their disease severity – perceptions of disease severity as well as actual disease severity need to be acknowledged;
- their previous experience of illness and knowledge of the illness (Davies 2008).

We have devoted much of this chapter to discussing the research ethics committee because without their approval you will not be able to start your research study. However, before you can commence, you also need to gain approval from the research and development committees/departments at all the sites in which you wish to conduct your research, so we shall complete this chapter by looking at what is required for research approval from these people.

Research governance

Research governance is the term given to the management, standards of conduct, processes and systems related to research. It is not a single process – many activities and concepts are found within it (Central Manchester University Hospital 2008).

The Research Governance Framework outlines standards and principles that apply to all research in the UK (Department of Health 2005), and an overview of the document. It:

- sets out the principles, requirements and standards for research at that site;
- defines the mechanisms to deliver them;
- describes the monitoring and assessment arrangements necessary;
- improves research and safeguards the public by:
  - enhancing ethical awareness and scientific quality,
  - promoting good practice,
  - reducing adverse incidents and ensuring lessons are learned,
  - forestalling poor performance and misconduct

(Department of Health 2005: 1).

Research and development approval

The Research Governance Framework stipulates that all research undertaken within the UK National Health Service (NHS) must have R&D management approval from the NHS organisation hosting the research before it commences.

R&D approval involves a number of elements, including:

- an assessment of the quality of the proposal;

- approval from a research ethics committee, ensuring that the project has received a favourable opinion from a research ethics committee;
- the resources needed for the study to be successfully carried out have been addressed by the researcher/research team;
- registration on the R&D database at the host site;
- honorary or substantive contracts with the hosting organisation for all the researchers involved in the research study (researchers with no contractual relationship with the NHS require an honorary contract. An honorary contract sets out the terms on which the researcher may conduct research in an NHS organisation and reflects the conditions which the organisation seek to impose and the ways in which issues arising will be addressed. Researchers with a substantive employment contract with one NHS organisation do not need an honorary research contract to undertake research in another NHS organisation – National Institute for Health Research 2009);
- Criminal Records Bureau checks have been carried out on all the potential researchers involved in the study and no problems have emerged as a result – this is a mandatory requirement for all research involving patients and clients (i.e. vulnerable people);
- support from relevant departments/mangers in the host organisation;
- research agreements with external bodies if appropriate (e.g. universities, patient organisations);
- research sponsorship has been addressed – and obtained if it is necessary to undertake the research (this is linked to resources above).

(Department of Health 2005).

Summary

In this chapter, we have introduced you to ethics and have highlighted some of the violations of ethical considerations in research studies that occurred in the past. We have also discussed the importance of ethics to your research proposal and to the study itself, have explained why research ethics approval is important and how you can seek ethics approval for your own research study. Points to bear in mind when submitting a proposal to the ethics committee are also addressed. It has been pointed out how the research framework provides some assurance on the conduct of your own and other research. Finally, we have mentioned the importance of R&D departments and that, in addition to receiving a favourable ethics opinion, R&D approval is needed from the (NHS) site where the study will take place.

Activity

All control trials are fundamentally unethical as patients are treated unequally. In the case where a treatment is advantageous, the control group is denied a potential benefit. In the case where a treatment is disadvantageous, the active group is exposed to risk. We cannot obtain truly informed consent from the patients because we do not know in advance the nature of the risk (Altman 1980).

- What are the ethical principles raised in this argument?
- Do you agree with the argument made? Give reasons for your answer.
- On what ethical grounds can RCT be justified?
- How would you feel if you were asked to participate in a RCT?
- Would the ground you have identified convince you to take part or not? Why?

Obtain an ethics application form. Complete as much of it as possible using the research question you formulated earlier.

References and further reading

Aita M. & Richer M-C. (2005) Essentials of research ethics for healthcare professionals. *Nursing and Health Sciences* 7: 119–125

Altman D. (1980) Statistics and ethics in medical research: misuse of statistics is unethical. *British Medical Journal* **281**: 1267–1269.

Beauchamp T. L. & Childress J. F. (2001) *Principles in biomedical ethics* (5th edition). Oxford: Oxford University Press.

Belmont Report (1979) *The national commission for the protection of human subjects of biomedical and behavioural research*. Washington, DC: Department of Health Education and Welfare.

Bristol Royal Infirmary Report (2001) *Final report summary and recommendations*. London: The Stationery Office.

Central Manchester University Hospital (2008) *Research governance information*. Hertfordshire: Brand Attention.

Chartered Society of Physiotherapy (2001) *Research ethics and ethics committee*. London: Chartered Society of Physiotherapy.

Collins Paperback English Dictionary (1986) London: Collins.

Davies H. (2008) Research ethics. In S. Porter (Ed.) *First steps in research: A pocketbook for healthcare students* (pp. 121–156). Edinburgh: Churchill Livingstone/Elsevier.

Department of Health (2005) *Research governance framework for health and social care* (2nd edition). London: DH.

Dubois M. (2005) Palliative and pain medicine: Improving care for patients with serious illness. *Techniques in Regional Anesthesia and Pain Management* **9**(3) (July): 133–138.

Fry S. & Johnstone M-J. (2008) *Ethics in nursing practice* (3rd edition). Hoboken, NJ: John Wiley & Sons.

Gelling L. (1999) Ethical principles in healthcare research. *Nursing Standard* **13(36)**: 39–42.

Gillon R. (1994) Medical ethics: four principles plus attention to scope. *British Medical Journal* **309**: 184–188.

Houser J. (2008) *Nursing research: reading, using and creating evidence*. Sudbury, MA: Jones & Bartlett.

Integrated Research Application System (2008) www.myresearchproject.org. uk

Khan J. P., Mastroianni A. C. & Sugarman (1998) Changing claims about justice in research: An introduction and overview. In J. P. Kahn, A. C. Mastroianni & J. Sugarman (Eds.) *Beyond consent. Seeking justice in research* (pp. 1–10). New York: Oxford University Press.

National Institute for Health Research (2009) *Research in the NHS – HR good practice resource pack* (version 1.1). London: National Institute for Health Research.

National Patient Safety Agency (2007) *Guidance for applicants to the national research ethics service*. London: NPSA.

Nursing and Midwifery Council (2004) *The NMC code of professional conduct: standards for conduct, performance and ethics*. London: NMC.

Parahoo K. (2006) *Nursing research: principles, process and issues*. Basingstoke: Palgrave Macmillan.

Polit D. F. & Beck C. T. (2004) *Nursing research: Principles and practice*. Philadelphia: Lippincott Williams & Wilkins.

Polit D. F. & Beck C. T (2008) *Generating and assessing evidence for nursing practice* (8th edition). Philadelphia: Lippincott Williams & Wilkins.

Polit D. F., Beck C. T. & Hungler B. P. (2001) *Essentials of nursing research: Methods, appraisal, and utilization* (5th edition). Philadelphia: Lippincott.

Porter B. F. (2000) *The good life: Alternatives in ethics*. Lanham, MD: Rowman & Littlefield.

Report of the Royal Liverpool Children's Enquiry (2001) *Main report and evidence*. London: The Stationery Office.

Royal College of Nursing (2007) *Research ethics: RCN guidance for nurses*. London: RCN.

Silverman H. (2007) Ethical issues during conduct of clinical trials. *The Proceedings of the American Thoracic Society*. **4**: 180–184.

Singer P. (1993) *Practical ethics* (2nd edition). Cambridge: Cambridge University Press.

Storch J., Rodney P. & Starzomski R. (2004) *Towards a moral horizon: Nursing ethics for leadership and practice*. Toronto: Pearson/Prentice Hall.

World Medical Association (1964) *Declaration of Helsinki: ethical principles for medical research involving human subjects*. Helsinki: WMA.

World Medical Association (2008) *The handbook of the world medical association policy*. Paris: Ferney-Voltaire.

The Research Proposal: Selecting Participants

Introduction

If you have been reading this book alongside working through the web program, by now you will have decided on your research method and your research question(s) and/or hypothesis. Now it is time to start to plan your research in detail and one of the first things that you will need to sort out is the sample for your research study.

This chapter, and the sample section in the web program, discuss what a sample is and how you can obtain the most appropriate one for your research.

What is a sample?

As you learned in chapter 5, a sample is a group of people who have been selected to act as representatives of a population as a whole. A population in terms of a research study consists of the people who may be affected by the phenomenon that you are investigating (e.g. people with HIV and drug dependency in the UK). The sample that you choose has to be large enough to allow you to investigate fully the phenomenon that is of interest to you using the research methodology that you think will best answer the research question/problem or prove/disprove your hypothesis.

According to Neutens & Rubinson (2002: 140): 'A knowledgeable researcher commences with a population and works down to a sample.' In other words, you select the population you wish to study and then derive your sample from that population rather than obtain your sample and then decide what the population will be. If you work out your sample first, you may find that it is not representative of the population that you are interested in (e.g. recruiting a sample of university undergraduates and then looking at the incidence and treatment of bipolar disorder or obesity among them and extrapolating your findings to the total UK population). So, it is important to determine your population and then settle on your sample, which should be as representative of that population as possible.

Why use a sample?

The simple answer is that it saves you time and money. For example, if you are interested in looking at an aspect of patients with diabetes mellitus living in the UK, you would find it almost impossible to study this with any accuracy in such a large number of people. It would be very expensive to contact everyone with diabetes mellitus in the UK and extremely time-consuming (Polit & Hungler 1999).

However, there are other reasons for using a sample than time and money alone. The possibility of achieving a much better response rate from a sample as opposed to a response rate from a population is greatly increased by limiting it to fewer people. The advantage of a good response rate is that it tends to make the results more accurate and valid, assuming your sample is truly representative of the population.

Certainly, in qualitative research where, for example, you may wish to do one-to-one interviewing, using a sample makes such research possible. This would not be the case if you were to attempt to interview a whole population. Whilst interviewing a whole population is feasible, you would need to recruit many interviewers, and this would certainly increase the costs and at the same time increase the problem of standardising the interviews.

We have mentioned above the importance of the representativeness of your sample. This is particularly important when considering quantitative research. So what do we mean by sample representativeness? According to Telhaj et al. (2004: 1), 'representativeness expresses the degree to which sample data accurately and precisely represents a characteristic of a population's parameter variations at a sampling point.' In simple terms, by representativeness we mean that we want the sample to have all the qualities and aspects of our population, and that means that the sample must include the same differences as are found in the population as a whole. For example, if we wish to investigate the effects on health of instituting a regime of a set type and amount of exercise with the elderly in Lancashire, we would need to look at the whole population of Lancashire and then look at the variation within the elderly population of Lancashire – age range, ethnic/racial percentages and gender populations. We would then try to ensure that our sample includes the same variations in the same proportions.

One of the main purposes of sample representativeness is to eliminate bias – hence its importance in quantitative research because it is essential in such research that bias is eliminated, whereas in qualitative research, where representativeness is not always the goal, any bias is acknowledged and is not so much a concern. Such biases can arise, for example, from a sample which does not truly represent the participant population (Telhaj et al. 2004).

There are other forms of bias, such as researcher or interviewer bias, but these are not concerned with the sample and are discussed in chapters 4, 5 and 8 and in the web program.

In terms of preventing sample bias, Telhaj et al. (2004: 1) point out that 'the representativeness criterion is best satisfied by making certain that sampling locations are selected properly and a sufficient number of samples are collected'. In effect, sampling bias occurs when there is either over- or under-representation of participants with the characteristic of interest to the researcher in the sample (Polit & Hungler 1999). For example, suppose you are interested in the quality of life of children with diabetes mellitus and you decide to undertake your research by taking a sample of children with this disease and asking them to fill in a questionnaire related to their quality of life. This is reasonable. But suppose you obtain your sample from children who frequently attend A&E because they have become ketoacidotic. This will bias your research because the sample is not representative of all children with diabetes mellitus, who are generally able to control their diabetes. (Of course, if you wanted to research the quality of life of children who attend hospital as an emergency because of ketoacidosis, then your sample would be fine.)

Probability and non-probability

Before we move on to look at different types of samples, a few points about two major classes of sampling methods that we use, namely probability sampling methods and non-probability sampling methods, are in order. **Probability sampling** is any method that produces samples that have been randomly selected. In order for your samples to be randomly selected, you need to have mechanisms in place that will ensure that the participants have the same chance (or possibility) of being selected. The simplest forms of random selection are picking a name out of a hat or drawing the 'short straw'. These days, we are more likely to use a computer as the means for generating random numbers as the basis for random selection.

Non-probability sampling does not have a mechanism for random selection, and therefore not all members of a population will have an equal probability of being in the sample. For this reason, non-probability sampling methods are usually not recommended for a research study if you want to generalise from the sample to the population as a whole. Although non-probability sampling is much less expensive than probability sampling, the results are of limited value if the generalisation of results is required. However, in many qualitative research studies, where generalisation of results is not required, it is in order to use non-probability methods to obtain your sample.

Examples of non-probability sampling include:

- convenience, haphazard or accidental sampling (see below);
- snowball sampling (see below);
- purposive sampling (see below);
- deviant case sampling – obtaining cases that differ substantially from the dominant pattern (this is a special type of purposive sample);
- case study – the research is limited to a small group with a similar characteristic, or even to a single person;
- quota sampling – here you decide in advance on a quota (for example, 30% made up of people aged 21–40, 30% aged 41–60 and 40% aged 61 and over) and then are free to choose anyone as long as the quota is met.

So now you know that the difference between non-probability and probability sampling is that the former does not involve random selection whilst probability sampling does.

With probability sampling, we are able to estimate confidence intervals for statistics (see chapter 8). With non-probability samples, the population may not be represented – or only weakly represented – by the sample so we cannot do this. Generally, however, researchers, even qualitative researchers, prefer probability random over non-probability sampling methods, as they are considered to be more accurate and rigorous.

However, in certain types of research, particularly in applied social or nursing research, there may be circumstances where, for various reasons, it is not feasible, practical or theoretically possible to have random samples, in which case non-probability sampling techniques can be used and, as long as a good rationale is given, it is usually acceptable.

Finally, it is important to note that even studies that started with probability samples may end up with non-probability samples due to unintentional or unavoidable characteristics of the sampling method. However, ideally we shall use probability samples, so let us now have a closer look at the different types of probability samples.

Types of probability sample

Random samples

As the term suggests, with a random sample the people who make up the sample have been chosen at random. The aim of selecting a sample randomly is to eliminate the risk of bias, and the principle behind a random sample is that each member in the population should have a greater than zero opportunity of being selected.

This type of sample is more usually used in experimental quantitative research designs rather than in qualitative research, although it is sometimes used in qualitative research.

There are different types of probability/random sampling. These include:

- simple random sampling;
- stratified random sampling;
- cluster sampling;
- systematic sampling.

In these the attributes of the sample and the population are a function of chance.

Simple random sampling

This type of sampling is the most basic of the probability sampling methods. Before undertaking this we first need to determine a **sampling frame**. Basically, a sampling frame is a comprehensive list of the members of the population that, as researchers, we are interested in. For example, to investigate a particular aspect of people who are assessing the diabetes services in a given area (i.e. your population), you would need to know the names of all the people in that area who are accessing the diabetes service. From these names you can randomly select an appropriate number as representatives of the population (i.e. your sample) whom you can invite to take part in the research. If we do not have such a sampling frame, then we are restricted to less satisfactory forms of samples which cannot be randomly selected because not all individuals within that population will have the same probability of being selected (Blacktop 1996). We would then have a non-probability sample (see below and the web program).

Once you have a list of all the population elements (e.g. people), they are numbered consecutively. You then need to select a method of randomly selecting the people who will make up your sample. This could be something as basic as closing your eyes and sticking a pin anywhere on the list of names; that person is then invited to be included in your sample. Alternatively, you could use a sophisticated computer program, or any method between the two. Consequently, a sample selected randomly in this way cannot be subject to researcher bias. Polit & Hungler (1999: 285) make the point that 'although there is no guarantee that a randomly drawn sample will be representative, random selection does ensure that differences in the attributes of the sample and the population are purely a function of chance'.

Stratified random sampling

This is a variant of simple random sampling, but in this type of sampling, before the sample is selected, the population is divided into two (or more) subgroups (or strata). The purpose of stratified sampling is to improve the representativeness of the sample. Put simply, stratified sampling is the process of subdividing the population into homogeneous subsets (i.e. each of the two subsets contain people who share the same characteristics, but there are differences between the people in the two subsets). From these two (or more) homogeneous subsets, the appropriate number from the population can be selected at random. These subsets/strata can be based on any number of attributes (e.g. age, gender, disease, medication) (Polit & Hungler 1999). One point to bear in mind is that your subsets may be unequal in size; in this case, you may wish to select your sample in numbers proportionate to the subgroups in your population. This is similar to quota sampling, a form of non-probability sample, and is composed of prespecified numbers of participants, who are included because they have similar percentages of specific characteristics of interest to the researcher as the target population.

Cluster sampling

Cluster sampling comes into its own when your population is very large (e.g. the whole country) and it is physically and/or financially not feasible to undertake your research on a sample drawn from all over the country. If this is the case, you may wish to select certain areas of the country at random (sticking a pin in a map whilst blindfolded is as good as a way as any of doing this) and then randomly select your sample from those areas only.

Whilst cluster sampling is far easier and cheaper than simple random sampling when you are dealing with a very large and dispersed population, there is, as Blacktop (1996) points out, a price to pay in terms of precision. If we intend to use cluster sampling in our research, we have to take into account that, as Blacktop (1996: 11) says, 'our political and social attitudes are shaped by the people we live and work with. Because of this, the people within a cluster tend to be similar to each other and to be different from people in other clusters.'

In cluster sampling, Polit & Hungler (1999) explain that there is a successive random sampling of units within the population, commencing with sampling large groupings (clusters), then sampling subunits within the larger groupings, followed by sampling smaller subunits within these, and so on. Because there is successive sampling of ever smaller units, this approach is often referred to as multistage sampling. It is important to note that the cluster samples can be selected by simple or stratified sampling methods.

Polit & Hungler (1999) note that there is a risk that cluster sampling will contain more sampling errors than either simple or stratified random sampling. Despite this, the method remains less expensive and is more practical than other types of probability sampling when your population is large and widely dispersed.

Systemic sampling

Systemic sampling involves the selection, not so much randomly as selectively, of every second, fifth or tenth (or whatever ordinal number you wish to use) person on a list. There is a formula for determining your sampling interval (Polit & Hungler 1999), and this is:

Sampling interval = population number divided by required sample number.

If, for example, you have a population of 1,000 and you want a sample of 100, then your equation is:

$$\text{Sample interval} = \frac{1000}{100} = 10$$

So you would select every tenth person on your population list. You then have to randomly select a starting point (again, sticking a pin in the list method is as good as any), so your starting point might be 12. In this case, you would select numbers 12, 22, 32, 42, and so on until you have reached the end, and then you would start at the beginning, so in this case your 100th participant would be number 2 because you have returned to the beginning of the list.

This sampling design can be thought of as either probability sampling or non-probability sampling; it depends on whether you select your sample randomly as above, or start your sample interval at number 1.

Types of non-probability sample

We now turn to non-probability sampling.

As a brief introduction to the different types of non-probability samples, here are some of the most common types.

Theoretical sampling

'Theoretical sampling is the process of data collection for generating theory whereby the researcher jointly collates, codes and analyses data and decides what data to collect and who to collect it from, in order to develop his/her theory as it emerges' (Ingleton 2004).

Theoretical sampling is the term used by Glaser & Strauss (1967) to describe the manner in which sources of data can be identified and then selected for inclusion in a grounded theory study (Benton 2000). The goal of theoretical sampling is completely different from probabilistic sampling (discussed above). Here, your goals as a researcher are to gain a deeper understanding of the analysed cases and from them begin to develop the analytical framework and concepts that you will use in your research.

In theoretical sampling participants are selected because it is felt that they can inform the researcher's developing understanding of the area of investigation. It is often used in grounded theory research in order to develop a theory through the research process itself. The idea is that the researcher collects data from any individual, or any group of people, who can provide the appropriate and relevant data for the generation of the theory.

In theoretical sampling, unlike other sampling methods, it is impossible to identify the size and characteristic of the sample at the beginning of the study as the sample size and characteristics grow as you generate more data until you have exhausted the source of new data (you have reached theoretical saturation), so, in effect, you can only identify your sample retrospectively once you have generated your theory.

Purposive sample

Purposive sampling (also known as judgemental sampling) is a non-probability technique that involves the selection of certain people whom the researcher wishes to include in the study. Participants are selected because they have certain characteristics that are of interest – for example, they have had the experience in which the researchers are interested or there are aspects of their lives which the researcher wishes to explore. In other words, the researcher deliberately (or purposely – hence the name) selects participants who, they believe, can add to the developing theory, support it or even refute the theory that is being developed to investigate the topic that is of interest, and hence is being researched (Ingleton 2004).

Convenience (haphazard or accidental) sampling

Convenience sampling (also known as accidental sampling) is a type of non-probability sampling in which people are included in the research study because they happen to be in the right place at the right time (Burns & Grove 2005). Put simply from the point of view of the healthcare professional, a convenience sample is a group of participants to whom the researcher has access – for example, patients/clients on a ward or in a clinic or the community, or nurses/other healthcare professionals in a hospital.

However, convenience sampling is considered by many to be a weak approach (but not as weak as volunteer sampling – see below) because it risks the introduction of bias. Indeed, to stress this, Burns & Grove (2005) contest that multiple biases, ranging from minimal to serious biases, may be found in convenience samples. This, accordingly, puts great responsibility on the researcher to identify and then describe any known biases that may exist. Once these have been identified, steps need to be taken to improve the representativeness of the sample. Transparency in sample selection and data collection is important in all research, but the use of convenience sampling greatly adds to the need for this.

In terms of sample size, in accidental/convenience sampling, potential participants are simply entered into the study until the desired sample size is reached. Thus there is no selection as such taking place other than that the participants are conveniently to hand at the start of the study.

Snowball sampling

Snowball sampling (also known as network or nominated sampling) takes advantage of existing social networks and the fact that friends and colleagues tend to have characteristics in common (Burns & Groves 2005). In a snowball sample, participants who are already part of the sample (often because of convenience sampling) are asked to identify others who may be suitable for inclusion and are likely to agree to take part. In other words, the sample gradually increases in size, like a snowball rolling down a snow-covered hill. This type of sample is useful when the researcher is studying a sub-group who may not easily be accessible by other means (e.g. drug users).

Another advantage of snowball sampling is that it can be an effective strategy for the identification of participants who are able to provide important insights, knowledge, understanding and information about the experience or event that is the focus of the research.

Volunteer sampling

A volunteer sample is one in which the participants have volunteered to take part in the study. This type of sample is generally regarded as the weakest form of sampling, but it is useful when respondents are difficult to recruit by any other means (see also snowball sampling above).

A major problem with a volunteer sample is that the participants may have volunteered because they have their own agenda or ulterior motives, which may conflict with the researcher's aims, so the risk of bias in the sample and within/between individuals is very high.

So much for how we decide which sample we are going to use in our research study. Remember that we choose a sample because it is often not possible to investigate a whole population. However, the number of participants that comprise the sample is very important for the reasons discussed at the beginning of this chapter. In the next section we turn to the sizes of samples and how we can ensure that we obtain the correct size.

The size of samples

Ingleton (2004: 123) poses the question 'does sample size matter?' She next ponders the question, if it does matter, how can we ensure that a sample is large enough for our purpose? She concludes that there are no simple rules we can apply that will inform us whether or not we have the correct size sample for our research.

There are certain types of research – mainly quantitative – where formulae are used to determine the sample size, and we shall discuss these later in this chapter. But whilst, ideally or theoretically, sample sizes may be determined with scientific principles in mind, in the real world sample sizes have to be achieved within the limitations that a researcher will encounter (Ingleton 2004).

Is this important? Burns & Grove (2005) believe that an inadequate sample size may well reduce both the quality and credibility of any findings from a research study. Similarly, in quantitative research, if your sample is too small, you may not be able to justify any generalisations to the whole population that you make from your findings.

The size of the sample depends largely on the aims and purpose of the research, as well as the current time and methodology used to undertake the research study (Merriam 1998). In terms of size, the main differences are between samples for quantitative research and samples for qualitative research. The major difference occurs because in qualitative research essentially we are concerned with the quality of the information that is being discovered, whilst in quantitative research the principal aim is often to identify relationships, causal or otherwise, between variables.

So we shall take these two paradigms as separate entities, commencing with samples for qualitative research.

Scenario

You are the lead researcher of a team that has been asked by a UK-wide charity to investigate the expectations of pregnant women opting for a home birth regarding their care and treatment before, during and after the birth, and then to find out if their expectations were met.

Obviously, you will be using a qualitative paradigm to underpin your research, but you still have to select the sample.

- In order to decide on your sample, what will you be considering?
- How will you arrive at your sample size?

Suggestions are found at the end of this chapter.

Qualitative research sample size

Burns & Grove (2005) make the point that the sample size and methodology of obtaining the sample are determined by the purpose of the study. This is linked to the depth of information and of experiences that are needed to gain insight into the phenomena under study. For example, in qualitative research it is possible to produce good research using a sample of just one person. Obviously, it is impossible to make any generalisations from this, but the depth of information and experience that can be obtained in this way can often bring insights that are of value to others. We often talk about 'rich, thick data' when we are undertaking qualitative research with small sample sizes. This is analogous to eating a slice of Black Forest gateau (qualitative research) which can be much more rich and filling when compared to eating a whole plain sponge cake (quantitative research).

According to Morse (1991) the important thing in terms of type and size of sample is the adequacy and appropriateness of the data that are gathered from that sample.

- By adequacy of data, we mean the sufficiency and quality of data obtained.
- By appropriateness of data, we mean the methods that we have used to select our sample.

This can best be ascertained when we are certain that the identification and use of participants for our sample can best inform us and help to bring insights to any phenomenon we are studying. In other words, our sample must do the job that we require of it.

Burns & Grove (2005) note that, in terms of adequacy, the number of participants in a sample in a qualitative study can be considered to be adequate when saturation of information has been achieved. Data saturation occurs when the researcher is no longer hearing or seeing new information from the participants. In other words, no additional data can be obtained.

Qualitative researchers, unlike quantitative researchers, analyse the data throughout their study rather than at the end of the data collection stage, so that they are able to ascertain when they have reached data saturation.

Important factors that need to be considered when deciding on the size of your sample in qualitative research are these:

- The scope of the study – is it broad and extensive or narrow and focused?
- The nature of your topic to be studied – is it clear and within their personal experiences, or difficult to define?
- The quality of the data that you can obtain from the participants.
- The design of the study – interviews, focus groups, questionnaires. (Burns & Grove 2005).

The scope of the study is important because if it is broad, then extensive data will be needed. This will entail adding to the number of participants recruited to the sample. On the other hand, if the study has a narrow, clear focus, then fewer participants will be needed before data saturation is reached. If the topic is clear, then fewer participants will be needed than would be the case if the topic is difficult to define.

'The quality of information obtained from an interview, observation, or document review influences the sample size' (Burns & Grove 2005: 359). Consequently, the higher the quality of data obtained, and the richer and thicker are those data, then the fewer will be the participants in a sample that are needed before data saturation is reached.

The study design is very important, as are the data collection methods used. For example, if the data are collected by individual interviews, then far fewer participants are required because the data collected are usually very rich and thick, whereas if the data are collected by means of questionnaires, then more participants are required because the data obtained by questionnaires cannot be as rich or as thick as those obtained by interviews.

Collecting and analysing qualitative data can be more cumbersome and time-consuming to record, manipulate and analyse than the analysis of quantitative research data. As a consequence, most qualitative studies take place using only small numbers within their samples (Ingleton 2004). This does not mean that all qualitative studies are small-scale; this depends on all the factors mentioned above.

Finally, it is important to be aware of your own time. Just how much time can you give to the research? Qualitative research can be very time-consuming and the data collection is not easily delegated to others because of the personal interactions and relationships that often take place.

Quantitative research sample size

In qualitative research studies, size is not a priority, although it is important that your sample is big enough for your results to be reliable and valid (see above). However, in quantitative research studies, size is everything. Lunsford & Lunsford (1995: 137) make the point that 'many clinical studies do not achieve their intended purposes because the researcher is unable to enrol enough subjects'.

Quantitative research studies, particularly where generalisation to a population is desired, require a large sample because if it is too small, then abnormalities can have a disproportionate influence on the results, and certainly more than they do in the case of the population as a whole (see chapter 9 and the web program). Neutens & Rubinson (2002) are very blunt about this and state that the larger the sample, the greater will be the representativeness of that sample to the population. Certainly, larger samples are needed when the population is heterogeneous (diverse), whilst smaller samples are generally satisfactory for homogeneous (the same or similar) populations (Leedy & Ormrod 2001, Neutens & Rubinson 2002).

Polit & Hungler (1999) stress that in quantitative studies you should generally use the largest sample possible for the same reason as that espoused by Neutens & Rubinson (2002), namely that the larger the sample, the greater the likelihood that it will be representative of the population. This is important, because every time a researcher uses the 'average' or a percentage based on the data obtained from a sample, he/she is saying that this is the average or percentage that applies to the whole population, so it must be representative. If a sample is too small in relation to the population, then an average or percentage calculation will be less accurate when applied to the population, so leading to the problems that occur with sampling error. It is to eliminate the risk of sampling error (caused by lack of representativeness) that we need to have as large a sample as possible and one that is representative of the population under study.

Power analysis

In order to be confident that you have a large enough sample for an inferential quantitative research study, we recommend that you undertake power analysis.

Power analysis is a statistical test that gives you the most suitable size for your sample in relation to your population. At the outset it is important to point out that unless you are proficient with statistics it is advisable to seek help from your statistics department when undertaking a power analysis. There are several computer programs that can do the statistical analysis for you, but you still need to enter the correct data, so recruiting a statistician is important even at this early stage.

Initially, you need to know which inferential statistical test you will be using. Examples include *t*-tests and ANOVA (see chapter 9). This will determine the size of sample that you need.

But first, we shall take a short diversion to look at the term 'inferential'.

Inferential

In this chapter, we have used the term 'inferential' in relation to research studies and statistical tests, so here is a brief discussion of what we mean by this term.

To give you some idea, the word 'inference' can be replaced by a whole host of words, including 'deduction', 'supposition', 'conjecture', 'presumption' 'assumption' and 'implication'. So with inferential statistics we are attempting to come to conclusions from the original data.

For instance, we often use inferential statistics to infer things about the population from the data we have obtained from the sample data. Alternatively, we can use inferential statistics to make judgements regarding the probability that a difference between groups in our study is significant or might have happened by chance.

In effect, we use inferential statistics to make inferences from our data to apply to more general conditions. This is different from descriptive statistics, which we use to describe what is actually happening with our data.

Inferential statistics are very useful when conducting experimental and quasi-experimental research design. A very simple inferential test can be used when you want to compare the average performance of two groups on a single measure to see if there is a difference. For example, you might want to know if a new treatment is better than the current treatment, and you can devise an experiment to compare the two – for this you might use the *t*-test.

So, when you conduct an inferential statistical test you are often looking at the difference between the outcomes of two groups or interventions

---

Another word that we have used in this section is 'power', as in power analysis. What do we mean by power in this context? Well, power refers to probability. In statistical tests we are often concerned with the probability that the results from our data have occurred by chance or are statistically significant (i.e. whether we can be certain that the differences identified are dependable). Another way of thinking about 'power' in this context is that it is the probability that the hypothesis or null hypothesis will be rejected or accepted. In statistics, it is accepted that you should have an 80% or greater chance of finding a statistically significant difference (if there is one), or to put it another way, the power probability should be 0.8 or greater.

Now another little diversion so that we can explore the term 'statistical significance' (which will occur in chapter 9 and the web program).

Statistical significance

It is possible that any changes/differences identified by your research study will be due to chance only, and if this is the case we discount any research findings as being unimportant.

In statistics, however, we say that something is statistically significant if it is unlikely to have occurred by chance.

We are very strict about the criteria for research results being statistically significant. This is usually put at the 5% level. If, from our results, there is a difference between two groups, then it is deemed to be statistically significant only if the probability of the differences not occurring by chance is 5% or less.

There are often differences found in our statistics, but unless they fall within the 0–5% range, they are not considered to be statistically significant and so are discarded.

We return to this in chapter 9.

Returning to power analysis, it is usually the case that the power of your test increases in relation to increases in sample size. Consequently, as mentioned above, in order to ensure that your sample size is big enough in relation to your population, you will need to conduct a power analysis calculation to ensure that your sample is the optimum size for your population.

There are four factors/values that you need to have before you undertake a power analysis calculation, namely:

1. The statistical test they you will be using (e.g. *t*-test, ANOVA, discussed in chapter 9).
2. The alpha (α) value (usually 0.01 or 0.05 – see below).
3. The expected effect size (see below).
4. The sample size that you intend using.

Having decided on these factors/values, you can then enter them into your computer program (or ask the statistics department to do this for you). Once they have been entered and the computer has done the calculations, you will be given a power value that lies between 0 and 1. If the power value is less than 0.8, then that shows that your intended sample is too small and you will have to increase it before you start your research. In fact, you may want to make the size of your sample bigger than is considered appropriate following the power analysis calculation because you will need to allow for attrition (i.e. you will need to try to estimate the likely number of participants who will drop out during the research).

Effect size

'Effect size is concerned with the strength of the relationships among research variables' (Polit & Hungler 1999: 291).

Even if you end up with a statistically significant difference at the end of your research, although you can be confident that there is a real difference you do not know how important that difference is. For that you need to calculate the effect size. For example, if you are undertaking research looking at possible differences between two groups, the effect size would be calculated by taking the difference between the two groups (the mean of one group less the mean of the second group) and dividing it by the standard deviation of one of the groups (standard deviation is discussed in chapter 9). This can become quite complicated, and as effect size can be calculated only after the research is completed, you will need to use an estimate for the purposes of the power analysis calculation.

To make this easier, a value of 0.5 (which indicates a moderate to large difference) is commonly used for the power analysis, so you do not need to estimate it yourself. Consequently, the convention is that you can put 0.5 as the value for the expected size effect in your inputted data for the power analysis calculation.

P-value and alpha level

The P-value is a statistical value which states the probability that the results obtained from our research study are due to chance alone. For example, a P-value of less than 5% (<0.05) means that there is less than a 1 in 20 probability of that result occurring by chance alone. It is considered to be statistically significant if the alpha level (α level) has been set by the researcher at that level.

Most of the time a researcher will set the α level at 0.05, so that any results that are greater than that can be discounted because the probability that the differences have arisen by chance is too great to be statistically significant.

Sometimes the researcher will be even more stringent and set the α level at 0.01 (i.e. there is only a 1% probability that the results are statistically significant). The setting of the α level is entirely the researcher's preference, but 0.05 and 0.01 are the accepted levels at which to set it. So, when it comes to doing the power calculation to determine the optimum sample size for your research, you would have to decide between 0.01 and 0.05 for the α value.

Sample size – continued

As you can see, the power analysis calculation is quite complex. Gay (1996) simplified the determining of the sample size for a quantitative research study by following four general rules:

1. When you only have a small population (<100) then there is not much point in going to the trouble of having a sample; it is better to use the whole population.
2. If your population size is made up of approximately 500 people, then 50% of the population should be sampled.

3. If you have a population size of approximately 1,500, then your sample size should be 20% of the population.
4. If your population size is approximately 5,000 or more, then rather than carry out a calculation to work out the sample size, a sample of 400 is adequate.

Although not as accurate as a power analysis, this is much simpler and a good enough guide, and is particularly useful if you do not have access to a statistician. Nevertheless, we strongly reiterate our suggestion: avail yourself of the services of a statistician if you are attempting *any* quantitative research!

Eligibility criteria

Once you have decided on the size of your sample, you need to determine whom you are going to include as well as who will be excluded. This is known as the eligibility criteria. When identifying your population, you need to be specific about your eligibility criteria. This will have ramifications for your sample, because, as you will appreciate by now, it must closely represent the population.

The inclusion criteria are the characteristics that people in the population must possess, whilst the exclusion criteria are the characteristics that they must not possess. When preparing for the research study you need to decide what the inclusion and exclusion criteria of your population will constitute. Polit & Hungler (1999) propose four areas when considering your eligibility criteria, namely:

1. costs;
2. practical concerns;
3. the ability to participate in the study;
4. design considerations.

For example, some of the eligibility criteria you may consider will include these:

- Do they possess the characteristics that you are studying – design considerations?
- What language must the participants speak? This has implications for cost (interpreters and/or translators), the ability to participate in the study (physical, psychosocial, travel considerations), design (interviews, questionnaires).
- Distance from your centre/home base – cost and time implications.
- State of health (physical and mental) – concerns over ability to participate and other practical concerns.

There are undoubtedly many more, but the eligibility criteria that you use to define your population have implications for the interpretation of the results as well as the generalisability of your findings.

It is essential that you give thoughtful and adequate consideration to the implications of the eligibility criteria for your research study. As Polit & Hungler (1999: 279) conclude: 'There should be a meaningful and justifiable rationale for all criteria that include or exclude people from the population and by extension from the sample.'

Summary

This chapter has discussed samples. The type and size of your samples are crucial to the accuracy and validity of your findings and hence of your research study. Because of the importance of correct sampling in all its aspects, if you are at all uncertain about how to determine your sample, seek the advice of an experienced researcher – particularly one experienced in undertaking research in your chosen paradigm. As this chapter has demonstrated, there are differences in the types and size of samples depending on whether you are using a quantitative or a qualitative research methodology to underpin your research study.

Now you have completed this chapter, and once you have worked through the appropriate section of the web program, you are ready to move on to the next stage – deciding on what data you want to collect for your research study and which tools you will use to help you collect them.

Activity

Choose a potential topic for a research study, Then,

1. Determine what type of research methodology you will use.
2. Decide on the size and criteria of your proposed population.
3. Decide what sampling method is best suited to your topic.
4. What will be your eligibility criteria?

Now make a few brief notes on why you chose the population and sample for your topic and justify your choices, particularly with regard to your eligibility criteria.

References

Benton D. C. (2000) Grounded theory. In D. Cormack (Ed.) *The research process in nursing* (4th edition) (pp. 153–164). Oxford: Blackwell Science.

Blacktop J. (1996) A discussion of different types of sampling techniques. *Nurse Researcher* **3**(4): 5–15.

Burns N. & Grove S. K. (2005) *The practice of nursing research: Conduct, critique, and utilization* (5th edition). St Louis, MO: Elsevier Saunders.

Gay L. R. (1996) *Educational research: Competencies for analysis and application.* Eaglewood Cliffs, NJ: Merrill.

Glaser B. G. & Strauss A. L. (1967) *The discovery of grounded theory: Strategies for qualitative research.* Chicago: Aldine Publishing Co.

Ingleton C. (2004) Populations and samples: Identifying the boundaries of research. In P. A. Crookes & S. Davies (Eds.) *Research into practice: Essential skills for reading and applying research in nursing and health care* (2nd edition) (pp. 113–128). Edinburgh: Baillière Tindall.

Leedy P. D. & Ormrod J. E. (2001) *Practical research: Planning and design* (7th edition). Upper Saddle River, NJ: Merrill Prentice Hall.

Lunsford B. R. & Lunsford T. R. (1995) The research sample – part II: Sample size. *Journal of Prosthetics and Orthotics* **7**(4): 137–141.

Merriam S. B. (1998) *Qualitative research and case studies applications in education.* San Francisco: Jossey-Bass.

Morse J. M. (1991) Strategies for sampling. In J. M. Morse (Ed.) *Qualitative nursing research: A contemporary dialogue.* Newbury Park, CA: Sage.

Neutens J. J. & Rubinson L. (2002) *Research techniques for the health sciences* (3rd edition). San Francisco: Benjamin Cummings.

Polit D. F. & Hungler B. P. (1999) *Nursing research: Principles and methods* (6th edition). Philadelphia: Lippincott.

Telhaj S., Hutton, D. et al. (2004) *Competition within schools: Representativeness of Yellis sample schools in a study of subject enrolment of 14–16 year olds*: Working Paper 2004/11. Institute for Education Policy Research, Staffordshire University.

Scenario – Possible suggestions

The first thing that you need to do is to determine what your population is – its location, size and characteristics. You can obtain this from the commissioning charity.

- The charity is a national one for the UK, so in terms of location, your population is found throughout England, Wales, Scotland and Northern Ireland.
- The size is difficult to determine, but given the recent increasing population of home births and the fact that the charity cover the whole of the UK, the population is likely to be quite large.
- The potential participants are obviously all women and all are pregnant. Because most first-time births are generally hospital-based, the likelihood is that the potential participants will be pregnant with their second or subsequent child, so they may be a little older than the average pregnant woman.

- You will want to consider undertaking a longitudinal study so you will initially contact the potential participants before the birth to find out what their expectations are, and then you will want to contact them some weeks after the birth, to find out if their expectations were met and ask, if they were not, what can be done to ensure that, in the future, they are met.

Second, you need to determine what your method of data collection is going to be.

- As the population (and hence the sample) will be widely dispersed, you may decide that a questionnaire is the most appropriate method because you can obtain data from more participants than by any other qualitative research method.
- However, you will get richer and more in-depth research by using methods such as one-to-one interviews (either face-to-face or over the telephone) or by the use of focus groups, although this will necessitate your sample being smaller than if you use a questionnaire.
- In the end, you decide that you will use both one-to-one interviews and a questionnaire – the rationale being that if some of the participants answer a questionnaire, whilst others are interviewed, you will get both rich, in-depth data and information from a large sample.

Now you can start to weigh up which type of sample is most suitable for your study.

- You will need two samples – one whose participants will be interviewed and one whose participants will fill in questionnaires. The interviewees can be recruited from among those who have completed the questionnaire. This avoids the risk of the two samples being significantly different, even though they both meet the eligibility criteria for inclusion. It also overcomes the time and costs of identifying and recruiting additional participants for the second, interviewee sample.
- You want your research to be considered rigorous and valid, and so you can immediately exclude:
  - convenience/accidental sampling;
  - snowball sampling;
  - deviant case sampling;
  - volunteer sampling.
- You also will want some form of randomisation in your sample, so that leaves you with:
  - simple random sampling;
  - stratified random sampling;
  - cluster sampling;
  - systemic sampling.

- You can exclude stratified random sampling because you do not want two or more subgroups that differ from each other, and systemic sampling does not fit your proposed scheme.
- However, you want a degree of purposive sampling because you want to choose only those pregnant women who have opted for a home birth.
- That leaves you with cluster sampling and simple random sampling. Both are satisfactory, but given the wide distribution of the potential participants, cluster sampling might be the more expedient for your research study.
- In the end, because you are using two methods of collecting data with two different samples, it is a good idea to use both cluster and simple random sampling:
  - Cluster sampling would be ideal for the face-to-face interviews because then you can interview representatives of the population in every region of the UK, so eliminating geographical bias and reducing the travel costs of interviewers.
  - Simple random sampling could then be used for the sample that is sent a questionnaire because travel costs are not involved.

Finally, as regards numbers – you will have to look at your resources.

- How much funding do you have, and how much can you allocate to the collection (and analysis) of data?
- How many researchers/interviewers do you have in your team?
- How will you analyse the data?
- What is your time-scale for the whole research study?

Only after you have made all these calculations can you determine your sample sizes, but the ideal is the largest number in both samples you can resource from your sponsorship money.

So you can see that, as regards qualitative research studies, determining type and size of samples is not a scientific process as it is with quantitative research, but is a logical process, often determined by other aspects of the research study, such as research design and data collection methods, as well as resources and the aim and parameters of the research study.

The Research Proposal: Collecting Data

Introduction

This chapter is linked to the data collection section of the web program.

> 'All research relies on data to underpin new discoveries or discussions of well-established trains of thought. Whether we term them data, evidence, findings or outcomes, they provide the reader with insight into a research project and allow us to critically assess the project itself' (Serrant-Green 2008: 3).

Now your research is becoming really interesting because you are at the stage of interacting with your participants, particularly if you are undertaking your research study within a qualitative paradigm. The data collection stage is crucial to the success of your research study. If you collect poor data or the wrong data, then your results will be meaningless or, worse, false. Importantly, it is crucial when writing your research proposal to be very clear about what data you are going to collect as well as how you are going to collect them.

Data collection is simply the formal term for how we gather information. There are many different ways of doing this for both quantitative and qualitative research studies and it is essential that you choose the method that is best suited to your needs. In other words, it must be able to answer your research question or allow you to prove/disprove your hypothesis.

It is also important to bear in mind that, as Cormack (2000) points out, no method of collecting data is perfect because every method has its limitations and strengths. Your role as a researcher is to select or adapt a method which is as near perfect as possible for your particular research study, and then you must be able to discuss the strengths and weaknesses of the method you have chosen as well as giving a rationale for why you chose it.

Once you have selected your data collection method, you will need to construct a data collection plan so that you can determine step-by-step:

- how you intend to collect the data;
- the sequence in which the data will be collected;
- the time and cost of collecting the data.

This will include the actual use of your data collection instrument(s), but you will also need to configure within your plan how much time you will require for:

- identifying potential subjects for your sample (see chapter 7);
- explaining the study to your participants;
- obtaining their consent

(Burns & Grove 2005).

Once you start your data collection – including the points mentioned above – you may find that practicalities will intrude and that you have to modify your plan. For example, you may find that potential participants need longer to reach a decision as to whether or not they wish to take part, or you may find that interviews are so exhausting that you need longer between them to analyse the data and/or to recover from the previous interview. Interviews can be mentally draining because you have to listen attentively, whilst at the same time thinking of your next question, trying to work out the direction the interview is taking or assessing if the interviewee is fit enough to continue, and so on. Depending on the subject matter, the interview can also be emotionally draining for both the interviewer and the interviewee; the interviewer later faces the same emotions when he/she transcribes the interview.

Another point that is very important to bear in mind when thinking about data collection is the importance of ensuring its consistency, particularly in research studies where there is interaction between the researcher and the participants (Burns & Grove 2005). If more than one person is going to take on the role of data collector (e.g. interviewer), it is important to ensure that there is consistency between them as regards interviewing technique, questions asked and approach to participants. This is known as **interrater reliability**. In addition, it is important that all the data collectors receive the same information about your research study, that they are familiar with the data collection instruments you are using and that they have received adequate and equal training (Burns & Grove 2005).

Collecting data

One way of characterising the differences between quantitative and qualitative research is by means of the methods that we use (Dodd 2008). In essence, methods of obtaining data for quantitative research studies include tests/experiments and questionnaires, as well as an examination of existing databases (electronic or otherwise). Whereas, methods of obtaining data for qualitative research include interviewing, observations and focus group work (Dodd 2008).

No matter what type of research is being carried out, all researchers need to think about (and later perform during the conduct of the actual study) four tasks concerning the process of data collection when writing the research proposal. These are:

- selecting the subjects;
- collecting data consistently;
- maintaining research controls – criteria of sample participants, methodological controls, elimination/admission of bias;
- solving problems/conflicts that may arise and jeopardise your study throughout the duration of the research project

(Burns & Grove 2005).

If you have been lucky with the design of your research study, you may have decided to use an established data collection instrument (there are many available for both quantitative and qualitative research studies). However, you may not find something that is suitable for your particular research study, in which case you may decide to develop your own data collection instrument. If you do, it is very important that you test it rigorously, systematically and honestly before the study begins. This will enable you to determine whether the instrument can collect the data you require. In addition, it will allow you to identify any parts that are difficult for participants to understand and/or to answer.

Another benefit of pre-testing your data collection instrument is that it allows you to estimate how long it will take to collect the data using that instrument, which, of course, has a bearing on the time allowance in your data collection plan. In fact, for this very reason, it is often considered a good idea to pre-test all the data collection instruments that you may be using (Polit & Hungler 1999).

So, now it is time for us to look at the selection of data collection instruments and methods for use in both the quantitative and qualitative research paradigms.

Quantitative research – data collection

'The fundamental principles guiding data collection in quantitative research are that data are derived in a way that is independent of the expectations of the observer and that the data are true representations of a phenomenon' (Botti & Endacott 2005: 188).

According to Botti & Endacott (2005) there are just two approaches to answering quantitative research questions, namely:

- descriptive; and
- experimental.

Descriptive quantitative research is concerned with the observation of phenomena that occur without any interference on the part of the researcher – there is no manipulation of the observed phenomena. Experimental quantitative research, on the other hand, is concerned with the manipulation of phenomena in order to observe the effects that this manipulation or interference has on other phenomena.

The methods of data collection for both types of quantitative research have many similarities. In theoretical terms, quantitative data collection is underscored by four principles:

1. empiricism;
2. measurement;
3. replicability;
4. objectivity.

Empiricism is observation and measurement – and whatever is observed or measured must be able to be replicated by others. Replicability is important because it ensures that any results found in the research can be repeated in replication studies by other researchers. Measurement requires the explicit definition of data collection tools and of instruments that have been used to measure the phenomena, whilst objectivity is essential in order to eliminate any biases arising in the data collection and interpretation (Botti & Endacott 2005).

In practice, there is a variety of techniques that can be used to collect data in a quantitative research study. However, all of them are geared to numerical collection.

These numerical data can be collected by means of:

1. observation;
2. interview;
3. questionnaires;
4. scales;
5. physiological measurement.

In quantitative research, the data are collected and recorded systematically, and these are then organised so that they can be entered into a computer database (Burns & Grove 2005).

Variables

The term 'variable' occurs at several points in this and previous chapters and is a very important element of quantitative research, so before we turn to the different data collection methods, a few words about variables are in order, because these are often what are being measured during the collection of data, particularly when using scales and other physiological measurements in experimental research.

When you look at many experimental quantitative research studies you will find that the phenomenon of interest is linked to various differences between people or within people, both before and after certain events or treatments. This phenomenon is what we call a 'variable'. There are two types of variables that we use in quantitative research, namely:

- independent variables;
- dependent variables.

An independent variable is the experimental factor in the research study that is manipulated by the researcher, whilst the dependent variable is what is being studied to see if the experimental factor has had any effect (Lanoë 2002). For example, if you want to study the effects of two ways of reducing a high temperature in a baby (e.g. tepid sponging and anti-pyretic drug) in order to see which is the more effective, then the different ways of trying to reduce temperature would be the independent variables, and the rate of reduction of temperature would be the dependent variable (i.e. it is dependent on the effectiveness of the independent variables).

Observation

In quantitative research, the observation must be structured so that there is a defined purpose to it. The first step in structured observational measurement is to define what is to be observed. A definition of observational measurement is 'the use of structured and unstructured observation to measure study variables' (Burns & Grove 2005: 744).

Once the decision has been made as to what is to be observed, the next step is to decide how the observations are to be made, recorded and coded. Observations can be made in a laboratory or a natural setting, and each can give rise to its own problems. For example, a laboratory is an artificial setting and may alter the behaviour of the participants, either making them more constrained and inhibited than they otherwise would be, or giving them licence to overact and adopt a false persona.

Within a natural setting, the same problems of influencing behaviour can arise if the participants are aware that they are being observed. If they are not aware that they are being observed, then there are problems linked to privacy and ethics (see chapter 6). Making observations using a data collection instrument/tool can lead to varying degrees of structure that are imposed by you the researcher – for example, there may be an unstructured observation of interactions between participants (more of a qualitative study), or there may be a more structured collection of data by tabulating such quantitative concepts as frequency of an action or degree of response to an action or treatment (definitely a quantitative study).

Polit & Hungler (1999: 314) discuss a serious problem that can arise from the use of observation as a data collection tool, namely its vulnerability to observer bias. They detail a number of biases which can affect the validity and reliability of objective observations:

'• emotions, prejudices, attitudes and values, which may unconsciously colour what the observer is witnessing;
• personal interest and commitment, which may cause the observer to see what he/she wants to see;
• anticipation of what is to be observed naturally, which affects what the observer has actually seen;
• making too hasty decisions on what has been seen before all information has been gathered.'

Polit & Hungler (1999) conclude that it is probably impossible to eliminate observation biases altogether, but the aim should be to minimise them as far as possible.

In most cases, a category system is developed for organising and sorting the behaviour or events that are being observed. The categories that are to be observed should be mutually exclusive. The observer may use checklists as an aid to the structured observation (Burns & Grove 2005).

Checklists are techniques to indicate whether or not a behaviour or event/happening occurred during the observation. Usually the checklist contains a number of defined behaviours/happenings/events that it has previously been decided will be the units of data that the researcher is interested in for a particular research project. A mark is usually then placed against that behaviour, happening or event, if they do occur. Behaviour that does not appear on the checklist is ignored.

Interviews

Although interviews are usually associated with qualitative research, they can have a role to play in quantitative research as well. In the case of quantitative research, the interview will be totally structured, with the interviewee being able to choose a response (usually one word) from a series on the interview form. Often the reply can be a simple 'yes' or 'no', or it may be a number. Alternatively, the interviewee may be asked to choose one item from a list. These replies can then be coded and entered into a database for statistical analysis. The interview may well be linked to a checklist.

In quantitative research, an interview is often used in these cases because of the poor return rate of postal questionnaires and checklists.

Questionnaires

Questionnaires may seem to be an easy option for a researcher, but actually are very difficult to devise and use correctly. However, they can be useful for collecting data on simple and well-defined issues.

The design of questionnaires should be carefully planned and **piloted** to ensure that they provide:

- the required data;
- data that can be analysed and used;
- an unbiased response.

Questionnaires should ideally be developed from a pilot study (see chapter 5).

There are two types of questions that you can include, depending on whether it is going to be a quantitative or a qualitative questionnaire. These are:

- closed questions – usually quantitative;
- open-ended questions – usually qualitative.

Often, we are warned against putting 'leading' questions in questionnaires. All questions are 'leading' in some respect though, but some lead more than others. However, they all lead towards an answer.

If you wish to construct your own reliable and valid questionnaire in order to collect high quality data, you have to accept that this is a subtle and sophisticated art. It is all too easy to devise a poor questionnaire, but much more testing to devise a high-quality one, but it is essential that you do, because poorly designed questionnaires produce poor quality data. Lydeard (1991, cited in Mathers & Huang 2004) describes the steps necessary in the process of developing a questionnaire for use as a research tool:

- Define the area of investigation.
- Formulate the questions.
- Choose the sample and maximise the response rate.
- Pilot and test for validity and reliability.
- Recognise sources of error.

Hagerty & Patusky (1995) describe the process of developing a questionnaire that they went through in order to measure 'sense of belonging' through a number of steps:

- The area of investigation was defined by reviewing the relevant literature.
- The questions were formulated from a number of sources, including a literature review and clinical experiences, and statements by people who participated in earlier focus group interviews.
- The process of sampling and piloting was undertaken with community college students and clients diagnosed with major depression in hospital.
- A third group of Roman Catholic nuns were subsequently sampled.
- Details of how the response rate was maximised (e.g. paying respondents for completed questionnaires) are also given.

- A good description of how the validity and reliability testing of the questionnaire was established is also included, for example, a panel of experts assessed content validity, and retest reliability was examined through the studies with the three subject groups.
- Finally, some consideration was given to the possible sources of error in the whole process of developing the instrument.

If you come across a detailed description of how a particular questionnaire was developed such as the one above, you can have confidence in the rigour of the study. But it also gives you some idea of what you have to do if you are developing your own questionnaire, so our advice would be, wherever possible, use an accepted questionnaire, or failing that, to discuss what you want to achieve with an experienced researcher.

In any research study which has used a self-developed instrument for data collection, sufficient detail should be given to allow for an appraisal of how it was developed before it was applied in the study. However, what is important is that you recognise that whether or not a questionnaire is an appropriate data collection method depends on the research question that has been asked. Indeed, you should always ask whether the method of collecting data was appropriate whenever you come across a research paper or a paper describing evidence-based care. You also need to ask whether the research methodology the researchers used was the right one for the research question that was being asked. This is why it is important that the authors of a research paper state what the research question or hypothesis is at the very beginning of the paper, in order for you to be able to decide whether or not they are using the correct research methodology and method of data collection.

Finally, when you become involved in a research study yourself, you must make sure that you know exactly what your research question is (or hypothesis is if it is experimental quantitative research), and also that it is the correct question for what you want to achieve.

Summary of questionnaires
- Careful questionnaire design is essential in quantitative and qualitative research for the collection of good quality data.
- You should look for evidence that research methods have been piloted and modified accordingly.

Scales

Scales are a very common data collection tool for quantitative research studies because they lend themselves to the simple collection of data from a very large sample/population; they also give rise to statistics.

You now know that quantitative research involves numbers, and we can define the numerical values with respect to the following measurement scales:

- nominal scales;
- ordinal scales;
- interval scales;
- ratio scales.

Nominal scales

A nominal scale is a type of measurement which has only a limited number of possible outcomes which cannot be placed in any order that represents what are considered to be intrinsic properties of the measurements.

On a nominal scale, numbers are present in order to establish identity only (e.g. male or female). Nominal scales classify data into distinct categories in which there is no implied ranking. Note that ranking means placing objects, etc. in order – 1st, 2nd ... 30th and so on. In nominal scales:

- Values are assigned to categories, e.g. in a sample, there are 50 men and 39 women.
- The categories cannot be placed in ranks of 1st, 2nd, 3rd and so on.
- The numbers assigned have no intrinsic meaning – for example, you may give each of the participants in your research study a number (1, 2, 3, 4 ...), in order to make it easier for you to analyse data from your research.

Data that are collected here represent categories of a particular variable, for example, gender, where females could be categorised as '1' and males as '2'. These numbers have no numerical significance.

Ordinal scales

An ordinal scale is a type of measurement that classifies data into distinct categories. Here ranking (or ordering) is implied and utilised in the research study. In these scales, the relative values of data are defined in terms of being less than, equal to or greater than other data on the scale.

In ordinal scales:

- Numbers are assigned to categories that correspond to order/ranks (1st, 2nd, and so on).
- Responses on the scale can be ranked from high to low, or vice versa.
- The distance between the first and second category does not have to be the same as that between the second and third, or the third and fourth categories.

For example, you may want to rank the ages of participants in your research study, and you could do it as an ordinal scale with the nominal numbers (which are assigned when the participants are recruited for the research) below the ages:

21,	21,	25,	31,	32,	36,	40,	72	(years)
3	8	7	6	5	1	4	2	(order of recruitment to the study)

You can see that there is no relationship between the ordinal and the nominal numbers.

Interval scales

An interval scale is an ordered scale (i.e. placed in order or ranked) in which the difference between measurements is a meaningful quantity, but the numbering scale does not start at zero. This scale allows you to rank the items on the scale (e.g. 1st, 2nd, and so on), but also to quantify and compare the size of the differences between them:

- Interval scales have similar properties to ordinal scales, with the exception that the distance between the first and second categories and the second and third categories are the same.
- For example, an interval scale of temperature could be: 96.9°, 97.0°, 97.1°, 97.2°, and so on. Alternatively, the intensity of pain felt by patients could be measured on a scale of 0–10.

Ratio scale

A ratio scale is a type of measurement in which it is possible not only to think in terms of differences in scores (as in interval scales), but also in terms of the ratios of scales. This is probably the most common type of scale and observations of this type are on a scale which, unlike an interval scale, has a zero value, but, like an interval scale, has an equidistant measure. For example, the difference between 0 kilograms (kg) and 5 kg, 5 kg and 10 kg, 10 kg and 15 kg, 15 kg and 20 kg, is the same at 5 kg, but at the same time a 20 kg child is twice as heavy as a 10 kg child. So, on the same scale you can have interval measurements and ratio measurement.

- Ratio scales have the same properties as do interval scales.
- But ratio scales also have items classed as zero.

Likert scales

The Likert scale is the most commonly used scale in quantitative research. It is designed to determine the opinion or attitude of a subject and contains a number of statements with a scale after each statement.

The original version included five response categories with each one assigned a value. The most negative response was usually given a numerical value of 1, whilst the most positive response had a numerical value of 5. So, the mid-point would have a numerical value of 3 (Burns & Grove 2005).

Response choices in a Likert scale usually address:

- agreement;
- evaluation;
- frequency.

Below is an example of a Likert scale:

Statement: Eating a good breakfast before going to work is a good idea.

Likert scale

1. Strongly agree
2. Agree
3. Uncertain
4. Disagree
5. Strongly disagree

However, note that the use of the 'uncertain' or 'neutral' category is controversial because it allows the subject to avoid making an unequivocal choice of a positive or negative statement. Consequently, sometimes only four or six options are given. When this happens, it is known as a forced choice Likert scale (Burns & Grove 2005).

Generally, data collected using nominal and ordinal scales are considered 'discrete' variables because they are not overlapping (e.g. male/female; high/moderate/low temperatures) (Polgar & Thomas 1995, Botti & Endacott 2005). On the other hand, data measured using interval and ratio scales are 'continuous' variables because the data represent a continuum where, potentially, there is an infinite number of values (e.g. pain intensity) (Botti & Endacott 2005).

Physiological measurement

Most nurses deal with the physiology or pathophysiology of patients and use many different methods and tools for assessing physiological functioning. Physiological measurements often find their role within quantitative research as either outcomes or dependent variables. Polit & Hungler (1999) note that most nursing studies using physiological measures fall into one of five classes:

1. Studies of basic physiological processes of relevance to nursing care.
2. Explorations of the effect on the health of patients of nursing actions or medical interventions.

3. Evaluations of nursing procedures or interventions.
4. Studies that seek to improve both the measurement and the recording of physiological data in patients.
5. Studies concerned with the correlation of physiological functioning with health problems.

There are two major categories of physiological measurements: they can either be performed on or within the patient (*in vivo* measurements) or performed outside the body (e.g. blood analysis), often in a laboratory (*in vitro* measurements).

That completes our discussion of data collecting tools used in quantitative research. Now we can turn our attention to those that we use in qualitative research.

Qualitative research – data collection

Data collection for a qualitative research study is very different from the processes involved in data collection for quantitative research studies, mainly because 'the procedure for collecting data is not a mechanical process that can be completely planned before initiation. The researcher as a whole person is totally involved – perceiving, reacting, interacting, reflecting, attaching meaning, and recording' (Burns & Grove 2005: 539).

Qualitative researchers have many data collection tools they can use so we shall look at just a few of them, namely:

- individual interviews;
- focus groups;
- observation;
- diaries;
- drawings.

The major data collection tool for qualitative research is not included in the list above, and yet it is crucial to the success of your research. This is the researcher. The ability of the researcher to communicate with the research participants before, during and after the collection of data is the key to obtaining good data, and subsequently to completing a good and useful research study. This is supported by Serrant-Green (2005: 3) who states that

'communicating with others lies at the core of the nursing profession. Our evaluations, and the decision-making that takes place as a result, enable us to make sense of complex situations and the experiences of others. Taking the time to listen effectively, assimilate and evaluate the messages we receive from our patients, clients and peers are essential prerequisites to "doing the job well".'

She then makes the point that we need to apply similar skills to the process of collecting and collating research data.

Beyond the researcher, the type of data collection that is used in a qualitative research study is dependent on the type of qualitative methodology you are undertaking (e.g. ethnographic, phenomenological) (see chapter 5), as well as which data collection method will best help you to answer your research question.

Flexibility is very important in data collection for a qualitative research study because the research study (including the data collection) is continually evolving as a result of the data that have already been collected (see chapter 5). Questioning and observation will therefore be informed by the theory as it emerges. It is not a static process, but a dynamic one.

The role of the researcher in qualitative data collection is very complex, particularly so when it comes to interaction with the participants. It requires considerable skill, flexibility, reflection and stamina. 'For a particular study, the researcher may need to address data collection issues related to relationships between the researcher and the participants, reflections of the researcher on the meanings obtained from the data, and management and reduction of large volumes of data' (Burns & Grove 2005: 540).

We now turn to the different data collection methods mentioned above, starting with one-to-one interviews.

Individual interviews

There are several types of interviews that can be use as data collection tools in qualitative research. The three main categories that we use are:

1. structured interviews;
2. semi-structured interviews;
3. unstructured interviews.

Structured interviews

Structured interviews often require a simple 'yes' or 'no' answer to the questions. Alternatively, they may be questions that require a set answer or just a number (e.g. in answer to the question 'how many children do you have?').

Whatever type of question is asked, the important thing to note is that the interviewee cannot talk about things that are important to them; instead, the interviewer dictates how the interview will progress and what questions he/she wants answers for. There is little room in the interview for spontaneity.

Semi-structured interviews

Semi-structured interviews are in-depth interviews (and so are often called a 'conversation with a purpose'). They forge a path between the two other types of interview – structured and unstructured.

With a semi-structured interview, the interviewer and the interviewee are equal partners. Basically, the interviewer knows the areas that he/she wants to cover, but allows the interviewee the options of going down a different path and exploring alternative thoughts and feelings. The interviewer, however, can then bring the interviewee back to the subject under discussion by the means of prompt questions, before allowing the interviewee to explore that aspect of the research problem, and so on. It is very much a two-way dialogue. At the same time, it is important to maintain a balance between flexibility and control.

A semi-structured interview will include many open-ended questions, although they may also contain some closed questions (i.e. yes/no answers). In addition, there will be probes and prompts to tease out from the interviewee various strands of their narrative to complete the story.

Unstructured interviews

As the name implies, unstructured interviews are the opposite of structured interviews. In unstructured interviews, it is the person who is being interviewed who can dictate the content and progress of the interview. The interviewee controls the interview rather than the interviewer. The interviewer may simply introduce the topic/theme and then allows the interviewee to talk about the things within that topic/theme that he/she is interested in and feels is pertinent to their life at that time.

Advantages and disadvantages of interviews

All interviews have inherent advantages and disadvantages. If you intend to include interviews in your research proposal, you need to be aware of what these are.*Advantages*

- Interviews allow the researcher to use the participants' own words, views, experiences, feelings and thoughts.
- It is possible to use probes during an interview in order to explore issues that have been raised by the interviewee.
- Interviews may reveal issues that previously were thought to be unimportant, or were not even considered, by the researcher.
- Interviews can take place at a time and place that are convenient for both the participant and the researcher.

Disadvantages
- Interviews are time-consuming, not only in terms of the interview itself, but also of the transcription of the interview and the analysis.
- The quality of the data is highly dependent on the skill of the researcher and the willingness of the participants to reveal themselves (often emotionally).

- Interviews are a socially constructed situation, so that what is said, discussed or inferred must always be understood within that context.
- Sometimes, the participant may feel under pressure to say what she/he thinks a researcher wants to hear.

Interviewer conduct

Interviewing can be a challenge for the interviewer – nerve-wracking, exhausting and stressful. So, it is a good idea, if you are going to be conducting interviews, to relieve some of this stress by drawing up a checklist as an *aide-mémoire* of what to do and what not to do (Creswell 2003).

You still need to be flexible, because interviews are rarely straight-forward, but at least if you can work through a checklist you will know that you have not overlooked anything, and that can alleviate some of the stress. In addition, a checklist is essential if other people are under-taking some, or all, of the interviews.

To give you an idea of what a checklist might comprise (which you may want to adapt as an addendum to your research proposal if it involves interviewing as a data collection tool), here is an interviewer conduct checklist developed by one of the authors for a research study into adults requiring palliative care.

Interviewer conduct checklist

- Do check that you have everything you will need before meeting the patient:
  1. Copy of consent form to give back
  2. Interview guide
  3. Tape recorder
  4. 2 × audio tapes
  5. Spare tape recorder batteries
  6. Contact details for follow-up support/counselling
- Do check beforehand that the tape recorder and microphone are working (also check after a few minutes into the interview).
- Regularly check that the tape recorder is still working.
- Be polite – remember that you are a guest in their home.
- Be alert to any signs of distress from the very beginning, and do finish the interview immediately if that is what the interviewee wishes.
- Stress confidentiality.
- Make sure that you get their consent again before beginning either on tape (see interview schedule) and co-sign the copy of their consent once they have consented again.
- Read carefully through the first part of the interview schedule to make sure that the interviewee understands what is going to happen and consents to everything.

- Before commencing, explore processes/triggers for 'time-outs'.
- Once the interview has begun, use the main question to guide the interview, but do allow some flexibility if the interviewee goes off at a tangent. You can always bring them back by using a prompt or probe.
- Use prompts to introduce a new topic or for follow-up questions to pursue implications of the main question.
- Use probes to help clarify what the interviewee has said or to examine what the interviewee has said by using exploratory questions.
- Useful probes can include:
  1. Body language
  2. Silence
  3. Nodding
  4. Saying 'go on'.
- All questions should be clear and open-ended.
- Avoid double questions.
- Be an attentive listener.
- Make a mental note of answers or issues that you will want to return to.
- Give the interviewee time to reply.
- Do not be tempted to finish the interviewee's answer.
- Do not assume – get clarification.
- Do not divulge personal details about yourself – you are taking the attention away from the interviewee.
- Do not make comments about any of the answers that you get.
- Do not be judgemental, by word, gesture or body language.
- Do not ask leading questions.
- Look for non-verbal cues, e.g. distress, irritation, lack of understanding
- Do be careful to pace the interview. Some of the interviewees may get tired very quickly.
- Don't be afraid to take breaks, but do switch off the tape recorder when taking a break (don't forget to switch it on again if/when you resume).
- Ending the interview:
  1. Try to end the interview on a positive and completed note.
  2. Remember to thank the interviewee(s).
  3. Reaffirm confidentiality.
  4. Give the interviewee(s) time to come out of the interview mode.
  5. Do emphatically switch off the tape recorder so that the interviewee knows that the interview is over and whatever he/she says after that will not form part of the research.
  6. Explain how the information they have given you will be used.
  7. Don't dash off (unless the interviewee is tired or has other things to do). Spend a few minutes debriefing both the interviewee and yourself.
  8. If the interview has not taken place at the interviewee's home, remember to pay them their travel expenses.
- Do not be afraid to write down even minor points that you have to think about – it all helps.

Scenario

And now for something completely different – this time we are going to have two scenarios (although they are linked), and for these, you will need the help of friends or colleagues.

Scenario 1

In this scenario, you are an interviewee as part of a qualitative research study that is looking into reasons why people become healthcare professionals.

First, write a series of questions about what you think the reasons people might have for becoming a healthcare professional. Then rewrite these in the form of questions, as if for an interview, and after discussing it with a friend, ask her/him to interview you using these questions as a guide. If possible, record the interview because it will help you when you come to the scenario in the chapter 9.

This exercise will give you a better idea of how you should conduct interviews rather than if you played the role of interviewer, because this way you will become aware of what works and what does not work from the point of view of the interviewee, who after all is the more important person in an interview.

At the end of the interview, discuss with your friend what you thought of the interview and also what your friend thought of it. This will cover such things as how easy the questions were to answer and which questions, if any, you thought did not work or were unpleasant or embarrassing to answer. Also discuss whether you got answers that actually answered the questions, as well as other things from the interview such as the interviewer's voice (tone, loudness, expression) and general manner. All this will be very valuable when you come to undertake interviews for a research study, because you will have experienced an interview from the interviewee's point of view.

You can then swap roles, so that you are the interviewer and your friend is the interviewee to test if you can put into practice some of the points that you discussed after your interview.

Scenario 2

Working with the same questions that you used for the interview scenario, this time you are going to use them as statements in conjunction with a Likert scale (see above and the web progam). Remember that the Likert scale has five points labelled:

- Strongly disagree
- Disagree

- No opinion/neutral
- Agree
- Strongly agree

The purpose of this scale is that participants in a quantitative research study are presented with a series of statements, and then they have to say which one of the five points agrees with each of the statements in turn.

Ask healthcare colleagues to rate on the Likert scale the possible reasons for becoming a healthcare professional. Again, save the results because we are going to use them in chapter 9.

Focus groups

'Group conversations are a common feature of human interaction. Through them we find that some people share our views and experience and others do not. It is an important way to socialise, share ideas and learn about how other people think and feel' (Parahoo 2007).

Focus groups involve a number of people being interviewed together (unlike interviews, which are usually conducted with one person). Even though a focus group involves several people, it is wise to limit the number to 6–8, otherwise the group can become unwieldy and difficult to analyse.

When setting up and conducting a focus group, it is essential to consider the group dynamics – for example, will it include a natural leader, someone who isn't taking it seriously, is a troublemaker?

As with all data collection tools, there are both advantages and disadvantages to the use of focus groups and we list some of them below.

Advantages

- A number of people can be interviewed at the same time; therefore, it is less time-consuming than interviews.
- Because of its social construct, a focus group may allow for common experiences within the group to be explored.
- The participants may feel at their ease in a group situation.

Disadvantages

- Group dynamics are important and that can influence the quality of the data generated during the discussion.

- Some people may dominate the group and this can lead to the (equally valid) views of quieter individuals not being heard or even acknowledged by the dominant members.
- Some members of the group may feel inhibited about expressing themselves in the company of others.
- Focus groups are difficult to organise – how do you manage to get a group of disparate people together in the same place at the same time, particularly if they are in full-time work?

Facilitating a focus group

The researcher who is facilitating a focus group is often called the moderator and has a very important role, just as the interviewer role is in an interview. So again, before starting to facilitate a focus group for your research study, write a checklist of what the moderator will need to be aware of and do. As with the section on interviews above, here is a focus group moderator checklist. One of the authors developed the checklist for the same research study for which the interviewer conduct checklist was constructed.

Focus group moderator checklist

- Do check that you have everything you will need before meeting the patient:
  1. Copy of consent form to give back
  2. Interview guide
  3. Tape recorder
  4. 2 × audio tapes
  5. Spare tape recorder batteries
  6. Contact details for follow-up support/counselling
- Make sure that you have a quiet, private room, with no interruptions.
- Do check beforehand that the tape recorder and microphone are working (also check after a few minutes of the interview).
- Regularly check that the tape recorder is still working.
- Ask them to introduce themselves by first name only, and to try and remember to introduce each contribution with their first name (it makes it much easier to identify them when transcribing the tapes).
- Make sure that you get their consent again before beginning either on tape (see interview schedule) and co-sign the copy of their consent for once they have consented again.
- Read carefully through the first part of the interview schedule to make sure that the focus group members understand what is going to happen and consent to everything.
- Go over the ground rules with the participants:
  1. Confidentiality

  2. Fair play
  3. Each participant has as valid a point as the next one
  4. Each participant has an equal right to express themselves
  5. No disagreements/arguments to be taken outside of the group
  6. Role, rank, profession and grade are not important within the group, except for the insights they can bring
  7. The moderator's word is law.
- Stress confidentiality and that nothing that is said inside the group is taken outside of it – apart from the tape recording.
- Before commencing, explore processes/triggers for 'time-outs'.

Below is a conduct *aide-mémoire* on the role of the focus group moderator, which was developed for the same research as the one the interviewer conduct checklist was compiled for. This will give you some idea of how to conduct a focus group if you choose this as a data collection tool for your own research.

Role of the moderator during the discussion

- Begin with the opening question to get the group talking and feeling comfortable.
- Allow plenty of time for discussion around key questions.
- The focus group moderator should keep as low key as possible once the discussion has begun.
- The moderator should have a low level of involvement when allowing participants to explore ideas and concepts.
- However, there should be a high level of involvement when comparing new participants with findings from previous groups (the idea is not to go over old ground but to explore new ideas and concepts).
- Be prepared to bring the group back to the topic if they have strayed too far – more important in a group than in one-to-one interviews.
- Encourage reluctant participants.
- Discourage 'over-enthusiastic' participants.
- Be aware of possible role differentials and how these could affect the group dynamics.
- Act as a:
  1. facilitator
  2. controller
  3. referee
  4. listener

- Possible problems to be aware of and to head off:
  1. Participants have different ideas about the purpose of the group
  2. Silence
  3. Participants who will not join in
  4. Everyone talking at once – control the group so that only one person at a time talks
  5. Running out of time – not getting round to all key questions because of too much discussion (often of irrelevant points)
- Do explore expressed views and behaviour.
- Finish by summarising, switch off the tape recorder and then debrief.
- Remember to thank everybody for coming and for his/her contributions.

Something that will help you to run a focus group successfully and is highly recommended is to have someone running the group with you (e.g. member of your research team or, if you are a novice researcher, an experienced researcher). Their role is to help and support you, and at the same time be able to observe facial expressions and other non-verbal signs that participants express. They can also keep an eye on the recording equipment and ensure that the tape or batteries do not run out. After the focus group, they can assist you by discussing what they observed and help you to place the tape recordings within the context of the non-verbal gestures.

To Do

Gather a small group of friends and set them up as a focus group. Ask them to discuss a topic – on any subject, not necessarily your work – and get them to discuss it as a group for 10 minutes with you acting as the moderator (following the guidelines listed above) and attempting to keep them on track while allowing each of them to have a turn at speaking, but at the same time allowing the conversation to flow.

This is good training for moderating a focus group.

Observation

Now we can turn to the third of our qualitative research data collection tools.

'Observing others is part of everyday life. We observe to make sense of the world around us, to take action and to make decisions when necessary. There comes a time, however, when it is appropriate to investigate our subjective findings more closely and objectively' (Pretzlik 1994).

Observation as a research tool covers the continuum from being a complete observer to being a complete participant. The researcher must choose what to observe and when to observe it (this depends on the research question). The data are taken as field notes so none of the participants' own words are recorded verbatim. This is particularly used in ethnographic research, but can also form part of data collection tools used in other qualitative research methodologies such as interviews and focus groups.

Again, there are advantages and disadvantages to this method of data collection.

Advantages

- Observation allows for events to be seen in the 'real world' and is not dependent on others' second-hand reporting.
- Data can be collected over a period of time (longitudinally).
- Different 'events' can be sampled until a good understanding of the social structure/world is obtained.

Disadvantages

- The researcher is the main instrument/data collection tool; therefore, the quality of data obtained is highly dependent on the researcher's skills.
- There is always the problem of the Hawthorne effect/reactivity (see chapter 5), in which the others in the group may respond to the fact that they are being observed.
- It is very time-consuming.

Diaries

Sometimes, rather than talk to your research participants (e.g. in interviews, focus groups), you can ask them to keep diaries in order to reflect on the phenomena that are of interest. These diaries can be filled in daily, weekly, when the event occurs, depending on the criteria and parameters you have put in place.

If you use diaries as a data collection tool, you are reliant on a data collection tool that enables behaviour, feelings and experiences to be recorded close to the time that that 'event', situation or experience occurred.

Again, there are both advantages and disadvantages to using diaries as a data collection tool in qualitative research.

Advantages

- Diaries minimise the problems of recall because the events/phenomena are recorded (i.e. the data are generated) close to the time that they occur.
- Diaries are useful when data of a sensitive nature are to be collected and an interview might be embarrassing.
- Diaries are also a useful tool when observation is not possible.

Disadvantages

- The use of diaries places most of the responsibility for data collecting on the participant/respondent.
- The completion of the diary may be haphazard.
- The accuracy of the data collected in diaries is difficult to confirm.

Drawings

Drawings are usually used with children or with adults who have mental health problems, because these groups lack the sophistication and socialisation to make their drawings artificial constructs. There is a series of drawings that children or adults with mental health problems can do to explore their feelings about certain events or phenomena. It is important to discuss with the participants what their drawings are depicting at the time the drawings are actually made (Vickers 2009).

As with all the other qualitative research data collection tools, there are advantages and disadvantages with this data collection tool.

Advantages

- Drawings may be an honest depiction of a situation or feelings.
- Drawings are useful when the participant lacks oral or written skills.
- Drawings bring insights that you may not have considered previously.
- Drawings can be fun for the participants and may be perceived as less threatening than an interview.

Disadvantages

- The participant may be too sophisticated or socialised to draw the 'truth' that you are after.
- The participant may be too eager to draw what he/she thinks that the researcher wants them to draw.
- The researcher imposes their own meanings and constructs on the drawings.
- An inexperienced researcher may interfere in the participant's endeavours.

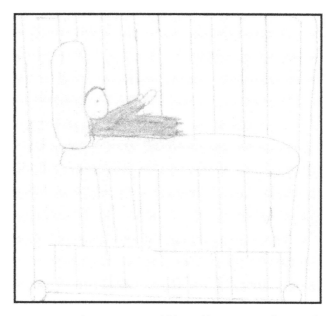

Figure 8.1 *Drawing by a nine-year-old boy of his time in isolation in hospital*
Reproduced with permission from Vickers P. S. (2009) *Severe combined immune deficiency: Early hospitalisation and isolation.* Chichester: Wiley-Blackwell.

Figure 8.1 shows a drawing by a nine-year-old boy taken from the author's research into the effects of early hospitalisation and isolation on children and families. It shows him alone, lying on a bed. He has drawn bars round his bed – an indication of how he perceived his isolation during treatment and to some extent his perception of his life at the time of the drawing (several years after he was in isolation).

Summary

The examples discussed in this chapter are the main types of data collection tools used in both quantitative and qualitative research. Other forms of data collection tools, particularly for qualitative research, include role play and other projective techniques.

No matter what data collection tools and methods (and even research paradigms) are used, the aim of data collection is to provide the building blocks that can be used to address the research question as well as to enable an evidence-based critique of the outcomes of the research study. Selecting the most appropriate methods to gather data for any study is essential to its success.

This chapter has looked at various data collection methods for both quantitative and qualitative research studies, and some of them, such as observation and interviews (albeit with differences in the actual use of the tools), can be used with both paradigms, although most tend to be restricted to one or the other.

One other point to make is that many research studies are neither exclusively qualitative nor exclusively quantitative, but are a combination of the two using more than one data collection method. This type of data collection and analysis is known as triangulation, or use of mixed methods. 'Triangulation' is the term often used to indicate that more than one method has been used in order that results in a study can in effect be double- (or even triple-) checked. (The process is also called 'cross-examination'.) It is hoped that by using triangulation you can have more confidence in the results of a research study if different data collection methods and analyses have all arrived at the same result.

'Researchers have a wide range of means of collecting data available to them, and need to consider which of these are best suited to their needs' (Cormack 2000). This chapter has attempted to guide you through the data collection methods available and how best they can be used so that you can be more confident of including them in your research proposal and study.

Activity

Think of two possible topics for research projects – one that is suitable for quantitative research and the other for qualitative research – then write down a hypothesis for the first and a research question for the second.

Now you need to decide which the most suitable data collection tools are for each of the two proposed studies. Give reasons for your choices and then make a list of:

- the advantages of your choices;
- the disadvantages of your choices;
- the problems that may arise and what you would do if they did.

References

Botti M. & Endacott R. (2005) Clinical research 5: Quantitative data collection and analysis. *Intensive and Critical Care Nursing* **21**: 187–193.

Burns N. & Grove S. K. (2005) *The practice of nursing research: Conduct, critique, and utilization* (5th edition). St. Louis, MO: Elsevier Saunders.

Cormack D. F. S. (2000) An overview of the research process. In D. F. S. Cormack (Ed.) *The research process in nursing* (4th edition) (pp. 63–71). Oxford: Blackwell Science.

Creswell J. W. (2003) *Research design: Qualitative, quantitative, and mixed methods approaches*. Thousand Oaks, CA: Sage.

Dodd, T. (2008) Quantitative and qualitative research data and their relevance to policy and practice. *Nurse Researcher* **15(4)**: 7–14.

Hagerty B. M. & Patusky, K. (1995) Developing a measure of sense of belonging. *Nursing Research* **44(1)**: 9–13.

Lanoë N. (2002) *Ogier's reading research: How to make research more approachable* (3rd ediiton). Edinburgh: Baillière Tindall.

Mathers N. & Huang T. V. (2004) Evaluating quantitative research. In P A. Crookes & S. Davies (Eds.) *Research into practice: Essential skills for reading and applying research in nursing and healthcare* (2nd edition) (pp. 95–112). Edinburgh: Baillière Tindall.

Parahoo, K. (2007) Focus groups. *Nurse Researcher* **14(2)**: 4–6.

Polgar S. & Thomas S. A. (1995) *Introduction to research in the health sciences* (3rd edition). Melbourne: Churchill Livingstone.

Polit D. F. & Hungler B. P. (1999) *Nursing research: Principles and methods* (6th edition). Philadelphia: Lippincott.

Pretzlik U. (1994) Observational methods and strategies. *Nursing Research* **2(2)**: 13–21.

Serrant-Green L. (2005) We need to talk – the role of interviewing in research. *Nurse Researcher* **13(1)**: 3.

Serrant-Green L. (2008) Data discovery underpins all our research work. *Nurse Researcher* **15(4)**: 3.

Vickers P. S. (2009) *Severe combined immune deficiency: Early hospitalisation and isolation*. Chichester: Wiley-Blackwell.

The Research Proposal: Analysing Data

Introduction

This chapter is linked to the analysing data section of the web program.

As well as describing how you intend collecting the data for your research study in your research proposal, you need to state how you will analyse the data. The problem is that 'raw' data on their own are meaningless, so before we can use the data, they need to be organised and interpreted – in other words, analysed (Botti & Endacott 2005).

If you have data from a quantitative research study, they will normally be in a numerical form; in order to use these data, you need to use statistics to analyse them. For many people, the term statistics can immediately make them panic, even mentally switch off, but in fact dealing with statistics can be fun! We all use statistics every day without thinking of it as statistics. The statistics we typically use most frequently are 'averages' and 'percentages' – as in the average age of the footballers playing for Manchester City is ..., or the percentage of girls who go to university to take a nursing degree is ..., and so on. So statistics are nothing to fret about, as you will discover as you work through this chapter.

Totally different from the analysis of data obtained from a quantitative research study is the analysis of data obtained from a qualitative research study. Here the data may be numerical, but they mainly comprise words, or sometimes non-verbal and non-numerical data such as drawings. In many ways, qualitative research data are harder to analyse because, unlike with quantitative research data which convert readily to statistics – and there are many different tests/computer programs to analyse the statistics for you – qualitative data analysis is less direct and possibly a little nebulous, as you will see. Although there are certain processes that we can use to help us analyse our qualitative data, the fact is that qualitative data are more open to interpretation than are quantitative data. Therefore, we shall start by looking at, and discussing, how we can analyse data from quantitative research studies.

Quantitative data analysis

First, a brief résumé of the types of data collection from chapter 8.

When we are undertaking quantitative research, data collection involves the production of numerical data to address the research objectives, questions and/or hypotheses. During this process, the variables in the study are measured using a variety of techniques, including:

- observation;
- interview;
- questionnaire;
- scales;
- physiological measurements.

Data analysis

What do we mean by data analysis? Well, data analysis is a process we use in order to reduce, organise and give meaning to the data we have collected by using the data collection tools discussed in chapter 8. Within quantitative research, the analysis of data involves the use of:

- descriptive and exploratory procedures to describe the study variables and the sample;
- statistical techniques in order to test any proposed relationships;
- techniques that will help us to make predictions;
- techniques that will allow us to examine cause and effect.

It is worth pointing out at that, unlike in the past, when dealing with statistics we no longer need to do calculations ourselves. Computers can perform most analyses.

The choice of technique that is used in any research study is determined mainly by:

- the research objectives, questions or hypotheses;
- the research design;
- the research instruments and how/what they can measure.

So, without further ado, let us start by looking at how we can undertake and analyse quantitative research, with a brief introduction to statistics.

Introduction to statistics

Always treat statistics with caution as well as respect, for as the British prime minister Benjamin Disraeli (1804–1881) once famously (or infamously) said: 'There are three kinds of lies: lies, damned lies and statistics.'

In this section we are going to take a general look at what we mean by statistics and statistical data. So, let us start with some definitions:

Data

We talk about data in statistics. Data (singular 'datum') are things known or assumed as a basis for inference, or, to put it more simply, 'Pieces of information that are collected during a study' (Burns & Grove 2005: 733).

Statistics

Statistics are concerned with the systematic collection of numerical data and their interpretation. Burns & Grove (2005: 752) refer to a statistic as simply 'a numerical value obtained from a sample that is used to estimate the parameters of a population'. The word 'statistics' can be used to refer to:

- numerical facts, such as the number of people living in a particular town;
- the study of ways of collecting and interpreting these facts.

It can be argued that figures are not facts in themselves. It is only when they are interpreted that they become relevant to discussions and decisions. So statistics are there to inform our discussions – they are a means to an end, not an end in themselves.

Sample

You may recall from chapter 7 that a sample is a group of people, events, behaviours or other elements you need to have in order to conduct your research study.

Population

A population is what we call the group of individuals or elements that meets the sampling criteria (a sample being representative of that population). So, if we were interested in looking at the number of childhood cancers diagnosed in 2006 in the United Kingdom (i.e. our 'population'), we might not be able to survey the entire population of children with cancer in that year living in the UK, and so we would look at a sample taken from all the children with cancer in 2006 living in the UK (see chapter 7 for the criteria we need to apply to our sample).

Parameter

Parameter has, like many English words, several meanings. According to the *Concise Oxford Dictionary* (1991) it can be defined as:

- a quantity constant in the case considered but varying in different cases;
- a measurable (or quantifiable) characteristic or feature;
- a constant element or factor, particularly serving as a limit or boundary.

You may be wondering at this point what this means in terms of research. Well, to simplify matters, let us look at the definition given by Burns & Grove (2005: 745): 'a measure or numerical value of a population' – in other words, the numbers found in any given population.

Statistics can be divided into two types:

Descriptive statistics

Description 'involves identifying and understanding the nature and attributes of nursing phenomena and sometimes the relationships among these phenomena' (Burns & Grove 2005: 733). According to Sim & Wright (2000), descriptive statistics have two functions:

1. organising, summarising and presenting numerical data;
2. describing the distribution (i.e. the structure of the data collected) which will help with the analysis of inferential statistics, which are much more complex (Botti & Endacott 2005).

Descriptive statistics include the presentation of data in tables and diagrams, as well as the calculation of **percentages**, **averages**, **measures of dispersion** (the variation or variability within the statistics) and **correlation** (the degree of relationship between two variables), in order to show the relevant features of the data and reduce them to manageable proportions. In other words, descriptive statistics involve the summary of the statistics in such a way that the researcher can organise the data in these statistics and give them meaning and insight.

Inductive/inferential statistics

Inductive or inferential statistics involve methods of inferring properties of a population on the basis of known results from a sample that is representative of the population.

To **infer** is to deduce or conclude from facts and reasoning (Shorter Oxford English Dictionary 2007), and inference is the use of inductive reasoning to move from a specific case to a general truth (and hence is also known as inductive reasoning). The *Shorter Oxford English Dictionary* gives one meaning of **inductive** as 'leading on to', and according to Burns & Grove (2005: 739), in relation to statistics, inductive reasoning is 'reasoning from the specific to the general in which particular instances are observed and then combined into a larger whole – or general statement'.

Thus, with these types of statistics, statistics are used to infer results from the specific study of a sample to a general statement about the larger population. So, inferential statistics are statistics that are designed to allow an inference to be made from a sample statistic to a population parameter. They are commonly used to test hypotheses (see chapter 5) that consist of similarities and differences in subsets of the sample under study.

These methods are based directly on probability theory. **Probability theory** 'addresses relative rather than absolute causality. Thus, from a probability perspective, a cause will not produce a specific effect each time that particular cause occurs, but the probability value indicates how frequently the effect might occur with the cause' (Burns & Grove 2005: 747); in other words, given a certain situation, behaviour or event, how often that situation, behaviour or event might cause a particular result.

So much for the general background to statistics; now we can start to look at some actual simple statistics. To begin with, you need to know that symbols are used in statistics to simplify their presentation. Some of the more common ones are given below.

Symbols used in statistics

As a form of shorthand, we use symbols instead of words:

- μ (lower-case Greek letter mu) = the mean
- χ (lower-case Greek letter chi) = each of the individual operations
- Σ (capital Greek letter sigma) = the operation of summing all the values of χ.
- n = number of observations
- σ (lower-case Greek letter sigma) = standard deviation (also symbolised by 's').
- x = mean value
- s^2 = variance
- SS = sum of squared errors

When you come to the statistical equations, you can refer to this list for the meanings of the symbols. Now, to boost your confidence and to demonstrate that statistics can be quite simple (and perhaps a little fun) it is time to look at some simple and common statistical calculations, which are regularly used in statistics – and to some extent in our everyday lives, although you may not be aware that you are using them.

Average

'Average' is a measure of central tendency and of location. It summarises a group of figures and smoothes out any abnormalities. It also provides a mental picture of the distribution that it represents. In addition, it can provide knowledge about the whole distribution. The word is often used loosely in everyday conversation; however, used in this way, it can conceal important facts.

There is more than one kind of average, so we shall consider these next, commencing with the type that we use most often when we talk about the 'average'.

Arithmetic mean

'Arithmetic mean' is the type of average to which most people refer when they use the word 'average', and it can be defined as the sum of the items divided by the number of these items. So,

arithmetic mean = 'the total value of items' ÷ the 'total number of items'

or in symbols:

$$\text{arithmetic mean} = \sum \chi \div n$$

Where Σ = the sum of χ (value of items) and n = number of items.

The actual mathematical equation is $\dfrac{\sum \chi}{n}$.

For example, if we were to look at the ages of child branch student nurses, a group of 21 students, in their first year the university, we might find that there are:

- 11 aged 18 years
- 5 aged 19
- 2 aged 20
- 1 aged 25
- 1 aged 33
- 1 aged 51

According to our equation, to get the arithmetic mean of the group's age, we add all the ages together (= 442) and divide that by 21. This gives us an average of 21 years (or 21.047619 if you used a calculator).

So we can see that the average age of this group of students on commencement at the university is 21 years. But can we now say that the age of child branch students on commencing university everywhere is 21 years? Hopefully, your answer is no. After what you have read in chapter 7 and 8, as well as in the web program, you should have realised that the group (our sample) is far too small for us to be able to generalise to child branch students everywhere else (the population).

To Do

Using the method and equation above, work out the arithmetic mean average age of your friends.

You should also have noticed that, even in our small sample, our average of 21 years conceals a very important fact: the great majority of these students are aged 18–20 years when they commence university; there are just three students in the group who are aged 21 years or over. Therefore, the average does not give an accurate idea of the group's age range, let alone allowing us to generalise. Always bear in mind the words of Thomas Carlyle (1840: 9) 'A witty statesman said, you might prove anything by figures.'

However, we do have a couple of calculations that we can do with these figures that can give us a more realistic average. The first of these is the median.

Median

The median, another type of average, is the value of the middle item of a distribution which is set out in order.

$$\text{Formula} = n + 1 \div 2 \text{ or } \frac{n+1}{2}$$

i.e. n plus 1 divided by 2, where n is the number of items.

Now we can return to the ages of the cohort of 21 child branch student nurses when they commence at the university, namely:

- 11 aged 18 years
- 5 aged 19
- 2 aged 20
- 1 aged 25
- 1 aged 33
- 1 aged 51

To Do

Use the formula above for median calculations, and work out the median of the group.

Remember that the middle point of the ages of the group when laid out in a line from youngest to oldest is the median.

1	2	3	4	5	6	7	8	9	10	11	12	13	14	15	16	17	18	19	20	21	rank order
18	18	18	18	18	18	18	18	18	18	**18**	19	19	19	19	19	20	20	25	33	51	years

Did you get the same answer?

You can see that the mid-point is the age at rank order number 11, which in this case is **18** years (as there are ten ages before that one and ten after it).

If we look at the formula $\frac{n+1}{2}$, then the mid-point is 21 + 1 divided by 2, or $\frac{21+1}{2} = \frac{22}{2} = 11$

i.e. in this case the eleventh age in the row, which is 18.

> ## To Do
>
> Now do the same calculation with the ages of your friends.
>   Is it different from your arithmetic mean average? It may be if you have friends of many different ages.

In our example, does the median age give a more accurate idea of the group as a whole than the arithmetic mean average does? I think you would agree that the answer has to be yes, because 18 years is closer to the age of the great majority of the group. However, it still does not identify the anomaly that is the ages of the older students.

So, we have yet another type of average to look at – the mode.

Mode
The mode is the numerical value of a score that occurs with the greatest frequency in a distribution. However, it does not necessarily indicate the centre of the set of data (Burns & Grove 2005).

> ## To Do
>
> Using the ages of our group of child branch students, work out the modal age of the group and see if you get the answer that we do.

Again, use the ages to work out the mode (remember that the mode is the number that occurs most often):

- 11 aged 18 years
- 5 aged 19
- 2 aged 20
- 1 aged 25
- 1 aged 33
- 1 aged 51

In this case, 18 years of age occurs more frequently than any other age in our group; therefore the mode of the group is 18 years.

   In this case, the mode is the same as the median (but both are different from the mean), but this is not always the case. Consequently, you need to look closely at any statistics, because they are not always what they seem to be.

To Do

Again, using the ages of your friends, work out the mode of their ages.

How does it compare with the other two 'averages'?

Finally, let us look at range.

Range

The range is an everyday method of describing the dispersion (spread) of data. It can be defined as the highest value in a distribution less the lowest. Let us look again at our group of child branch student nurses. The range of ages is 18–51 years. Therefore, the range of ages is 51 – 18 years = 33 years. If you combine this with a modal age of 18, what does this tell you about the general age of student nurses in the child branch?

Answer: with a modal age of 18, although there is a range of 33 years (from 18 to 51 years), whilst most of the student nurses are young, there are some older ones (and even one of 51 years), but most of the child branch student nurses are at the younger end of the age range.

To Do

Finally, work out the range of ages of your group of friends.

Now you can reflect on your friends, their ages and whether you have friends mainly of the same age as you or friends whose ages are very wide-ranging.

Does this say anything about you and your criteria for friendship?

So, you can see that statistics are not just a string of numbers and lots of calculations, but are a starting point for debate and discussion.

Reflection on averages

Often range is given along with mean, median or mode. Why?

Answer: the advantage of giving range and one of the averages is that you get a much better idea of the group's ages as in the example of the child branch student nurses. It also overcomes the problem of how we demonstrate that there are some major anomalies in our group, which are virtually ignored by the various averages. (The 'anomalies' in our example are the students who are much older than most of the group.)

So, we can say that the group of child branch student nurses has a:

- mean of 21 years
- median of 18 years
- mode of 18 years
- range of 18–51 years

and we now have a clearer picture of the group in terms of their ages.

Standard deviation

We just have one more important simple statistic to discuss: standard deviation.

Standard deviation is a simple measure of the variability or dispersion (distribution) of a set of data. Basically, it measures the spread of the data about the mean value. A low standard deviation is an indication that all the individual data points are very close to the same value (i.e. the mean – see above), while a high standard deviation is an indication that the data are spread over a wide range of values.

There is a formula to help us to work out standard deviation:

$$\sigma = \frac{\sqrt{\sum (\chi - \mu)^2}}{n}$$

The same symbol you were introduced to earlier are relevant to this formula. So this formula (in words) is 'Standard deviation (σ) equals the square root ($\sqrt{}$) of the sum of ($\sum$) the mean value minus the mean squared ($[\chi - \mu]^2$), divided by the number of observations (n).

For an example of how we calculate a standard deviation, let us look at the group of students (our population) we used above in our discussion of averages.

We want to find the standard deviation of:

18 18 18 18 18 18 18 18 18 18 18 19 19 19 19 19 20 20 25 33 51 years

First, we have to work out the arithmetic mean. We have already done this and obtained a mean of 21. Now we need to subtract that from each of the ages and square the result. So, for example, 18 – 21 = –3, and squared = 9 (minus numbers squared = positive numbers).

Score	Deviation	Squared deviation
χ	$\chi - \mu$	$(\chi - \mu)^2$
18	–3	9
18	–3	9
18	–3	9
18	–3	9
18	–3	9
18	–3	9

Score	Deviation	Squared deviation
18	−3	9
18	−3	9
18	−3	9
18	−3	9
18	−3	9
19	−2	4
19	−2	4
19	−2	4
19	−2	4
19	−2	4
20	−1	2
20	−1	2
25	4	16
33	12	144
51	12	900

Next we have to add up these results. (This is where a calculator comes in handy, and even more so for the next two parts of the equation.)

The total of the squared deviations is 1,183, which we now divide by the number of subjects (21), or 1,183 ÷ 21 = 56.34. Now find the square root of 56.34, which is 7.505997601918082 (rounded = 7.5).

This is the standard deviation, but what do we do with it? The 7.5 score that we have for this group of students is used to give us an idea of the spread of the data that we have regarding the age of the age range.

So if the mean is 21, first we have to see how many of the students fall within one standard deviation (i.e. 7.5) of the mean. In other words, how many students fall within the range of 13.5 – 28.5 (7.5 either side of 21). Well, 18 out of 21 fall between 13.5 and 21, whilst one falls within the range between 21 and 28.5. That means that 19 out of 21 (90%) of the student nurses fall within one standard deviation of the mean. Next we look at how many fall between 6 and 13.5 and between 28.5 and 36 (i.e. within the second standard deviation). The answer is that none falls between 6 and 13.5, and one falls between 28.5 and 36 (5%). Finally, three standard deviations would be ages between 0 and 6 and between 36 and 43.5 – the answer is none. The only remaining student falls between 43.5 and 51, which is four standard deviations. So, given these results, it is clear that, although the group is very homogeneous as regards their ages, there are two students who cause the spread of data to be extensive. According to Hinton (1995: 15–16), in many cases 'most of the scores (about two-thirds – about 66.7%) will lie within one standard deviation less than, and one standard deviation greater than, the mean'. Our group does not quite fit that finding, with 90% being within one standard deviation, however, there is a special reason for this, and that is that our population is unique in that student nurses, particularly child branch students, are generally starting out in the world after leaving school, and so they will generally be around the same age.

A word of caution – the formula works for a population. If, however, we wanted to calculate the standard deviation of a sample, the formula is slightly different, namely:

$$\sigma = \frac{\sqrt{\sum (\chi - \mu)^2}}{n-1}$$

However, the rest of the calculation is as described above, but with the final stage of the calculation using the denominator n – 1 rather than just n.

Summary

This concludes our brief look at statistics. All the statistics you will encounter are variants of these. Some of them may be more complicated, but, like the examples given above, all are attempting to make sense of numerical data.

Finally, a reminder to be wary of statistics when they are presented to you:

> 'He uses statistics as a drunken man uses a lamp post – for support rather than illumination' (attributed to Andrew Lang, 1844–1912).

Data analysis

Let us commence our look at data analysis by looking at a hypothetical research study.

There are different ways of approaching our research question/ hypothesis, and the way we put together our research question will determine the type of methodology, data collection method, statistics, analysis and presentation we shall use to approach our research problem.

Examples of research questions

- Are females more likely to be nurses than males?
- Is the proportion of males who are nurses the same as the proportion of females?
- Is there a relationship between gender and becoming a nurse?

In these examples, you can see that there are three ways to approach the research problem, which is concerned with the relationship between males and females in nursing, but the way in which the problem is expressed as a question will determine your methodology.

Another research problem with variables

Hypothesis

In Greater Manchester, fewer females per head of population smoke than do males per head of population.

Let us begin with a reminder about variables. According to Burns & Grove (2005: 755), variables are 'qualities, properties, and/or characteristics of persons, things, or situations that change or vary, and that can be manipulated, measured, or controlled in a research study'.

There are different types of variables, namely:

- **Dependent variables** – the response, the behaviour or the outcome that is predicted and measured in research
- **Independent variables** – an independent variable is the treatment, the intervention or the experimental activity that is manipulated or altered (varied) by the researcher during the research study in order to create an effect on (change) the dependent variables.

Changes in the dependent variable are thus presumed to be caused by the independent variables.

Having recapped, let us return to the problem. In this second research problem/hypothesis – the relationship between gender and smoking – you can see that there are two categorical variables (gender and smoker), with two or more categories in each:

- Gender (male/female)
- Smoker (yes/no)

In this study, you will be looking for whether or not there is any statistical significance in the results following the research study. To achieve this we need to use alpha (α) levels and their importance to the concept of statistical significance. We discussed this in chapter 7 in relation to selecting samples from populations, but α levels are used in research statistics as well, and this is what we shall be concentrating on here.

Alpha level (p level)

The acceptance or rejection of a hypothesis is based on a level of significance (see below) – the alpha (α) level. This is usually set at 5% (0.05), followed in popularity by 1% (0.01), α level. We usually designate these as p, i.e. $p = 0.05$ or $p = 0.01$. What do we mean by levels of significance that the p value can give?

Levels of significance

Levels of significance are concerned with confidence levels, and the question that significance levels are intended to answer is: 'How confident can we be that the results have not arisen by chance and are therefore significant and can be trusted?'

The confidence levels are expressed as a percentage. This is expressed by a p value, so:

If $p = 1.00$, then there would be a 100% possibility that the results were all completely by chance.

If $p = 0.50$, then there would be a 50% possibility that the results occurred by chance

If $p = 0.10$ …

You get the picture!

If $p = 0.05$, we are 95% certain that the results did not arise by chance, and if $p = 0.01$, we are 99% certain that the results did not arise by chance.

We want our results to be as accurate as possible, so we set our significance levels as low as possible – usually at 5% ($p = 0.05$), or better still, at 1% ($p = 0.01$). Anything above these levels we discount as not being accurate enough – in other words, the results are not significant.

Now, you may be thinking that if something could not have arisen by chance 90 times out of 100 (p = 0.1), then that is pretty significant. This may be true, but what we are determining with our levels of significance, is **statistical significance**, and we are much more stringent with that, so we would usually not accept anything greater than $p = 0.05$.

So when you are looking at the statistics in a research paper, always check the p values to find out whether the results are statistically significant or not.

Statistical tests

Writing about data analysis in a quantitative research study, Black (1997: 3) makes the point that 'a nurse researcher is likely to want to use the skills of an experienced statistician at this stage, perhaps using a dedicated software package, but should have a clear understanding of the types of statistical techniques that are appropriate to the analysis of the data which has been collected'.

We have repeatedly stressed that if you are going to undertake a quantitative research study with numerical statistics, you should try to enlist the help of a statistician or a researcher who is experienced and confident with statistics, but we also concur with Black (1997) that you should be familiar with the most frequently used statistical techniques so that even if a statistician does the calculations for you you will still be able to make sense of them, and therefore have a fuller understanding of the research study (and its results) that you have undertaken. To that end, we now turn to statistical techniques/tests.

There are many tests that we can use to analyse our data, and which one we use to analyse the data depends on what we are looking for, as well as what data we collected and how we collected them. This is one reason why, unless you are very familiar and confident with statistics, you should always seek the advice of a statistician or experienced quantitative researcher when you start to write your research proposal.

When it comes to the selection of the appropriate test for your research, in order to determine the p value, you need to base the selection on four factors, namely:

- the level of data (nominal, ordinal, ratio or interval);
- the number of groups/samples in your research study (one, two or more);
- whether the data collected from independent groups/samples were from related groups. (Remember that independent groups are two or more separate groups of participants, whilst related groups are often the same group, but at a different time in the study, e.g. pre- and post-testing, or even a different environment);
- the characteristics of the data – in other words, the distribution of the data

(Botti & Endacott 2005).

Parametric/non-parametric tests

The large number of statistical tests and techniques are classified into two groups: parametric and non-parametric. Parametric statistics are more 'powerful' than non-parametric statistics, but have far more 'strings' attached to them (Pallant 2001).

Because parametric statistics use the arithmetic mean in their calculations, the data used in these tests must be measured at the interval or ratio level (see chapter 8) (Botti & Endacott 2005). Parametric tests are used when several assumptions about the research are met:

- Scores in the population are normally (or approximately normally) distributed around the mean.
- Population variances of the groups are approximately equal and can be calculated.
- The level of measurement should be interval or ratio (see chapter 8).
- The data can be treated as samples that are randomly selected.

Examples of parametric tests are:

- *t*-tests
- Pearson correlation
- ANOVA (analysis of variance)

Non-parametric tests are used when the criteria for parametric tests are not met. In other words when:

- there are deviations in the assumptions, so no assumptions can be made about the population or the data itself;
- nominal- and ordinal-level data are the measurement used for analysis (Neutens & Rubinson 2002, Crookes & Davies 2004)

Because these non-parametric tests do not meet the assumptions required for parametric statistics, they are often referred to as 'assumption-free' tests. In addition, they do not use raw data (e.g. arithmetic means), but data that are ranked from the lowest to the highest score – the analysis is of these ranked data. Using this method, important information about the data is lost – hence they are considered less 'powerful' (Botti & Endacott 2005). In other words, it is less likely for any significant effect that exists to be found using non-parametric tests.

Examples of non-parametric tests are:

- Chi-square test;
- Kruskall-Wallis test;
- Wilcoxon signed-rank test;
- Mann-Whitney *U* test;
- Spearman rank correlation coefficient.

Knowledge of whether your research is parametric or non-parametric will be one of the factors in deciding which statistical test to use. Some are used when parametric statistics are analysed, whereas others are used when non-parametric statistics are analysed.

Common statistical tests

Below are a few of the more common statistical tests you may come across in research papers and may wish to use for your own quantitative research study. There are many more, but we are not going to consider them all in this book, nor will we go into any detail about the ones that are included, otherwise it could get very complicated – again, rely on a friendly statistician or experienced quantitative researcher to guide you.

Parametric tests

t-test

The *t*-test assesses whether the means of two groups are statistically different from each other. This analysis is appropriate whenever you want to compare the means of two groups.

If you only have one sample, it can be used to test the mean of the sample against a specified value, but with two samples, it can be used to compare the means of the two samples.

There are three types of *t*-tests:

1. one-sample – compares the mean of one sample to a fixed estimate;
2. independent samples – compares the means of two independent groups;
3. paired samples – the evaluation of two groups that are related to each other, e.g. data from a group of participants who are tested before and after a procedure.

Pearson correlation

We use the Pearson's correlation test to find a correlation between at least two continuous variables. The value for such a correlation lies between 0.00 (no correlation) and 1.00 (perfect correlation). Other important factors (e.g. the size of the sample) will need to become involved in order to determine if the correlation is significant. Generally, correlations above 0.80 are considered high.

Note that a correlation is a number between −1 and +1 that measures the degree of association between two variables (e.g. X and Y). If there is a positive value, then the implication is that there is a positive association (i.e. if X has large values, then so will Y, whilst small values of X tend to be correlated, or associated, with small values of Y). If a negative value ensues from a correlation test, then this implies the existence of a negative or inverse association (i.e. large values of X tend to be correlated with small values of Y and vice versa).

In probability statistics, correlation is often measured as a correlation coefficient and is an indicator of the strength and direction of a linear relationship between two random variables. A number of different coefficients are used for different situations, of which Pearson's is the best known correlation coefficient.

ANOVA (analysis of variance)

ANOVA is one of a number of tests (ANCOVA – analysis of covariance – and MANOVA – multivariate analysis of variance) used to describe or compare the relationship among a number of groups.

ANOVA is used to analyse the means of two or more groups. It is a generalisation of the *t*-test (see above) which can only compare the means of one or two groups.

Non-parametric tests
Chi-square test
There are two types of chi-square tests and both involve categorical data (i.e. data that use categories) (Pallant 2001).

The first type compares the frequency count of what is expected against what is actually observed. In other words, it allows you to compare a sample distribution of data with a population distribution that has been derived from a theory or a null hypothesis. From this, you can decide whether or not a sample could reasonably be accepted as a random sample from that population (Koosis 1997). This is often known as a one-sample chi-square. The second type is known as a chi-square test with two variables or the chi-square test for independence. As the name implies, it compares the frequency of cases which are found in various categories of one variable with those of a second variable (Pallant 2001). In other words, with this test you are exploring the relationship between two categorical variables (e.g. gender and smoking/non-smoking).

Kruskal-Wallis test
This test is used to compare the mean from more than two samples, when either the data are ordinal or the distribution is not normal. If there are only two groups, then it is the equivalent of the Mann-Whitney U-test (see below), so you may as well use that test if you have just two groups.

The Kruskal-Wallis test is normally used when you want to determine the significance of difference among three or more groups.

Wilcoxon signed-rank test
This is the most common non-parametric test for a two-sampled repeated measures design of research study. It is also known as the Wilcoxon matched-pairs test.

This test is linked to ordinal measures (see chapter 8) and makes use of an ordinal-dependent variable, ordinal continuous distribution and random samples (Neutens & Rubinson 2002). It is similar to a paired t-test, except that it is a non-parametric test whilst the t-test is a parametric test.

Note: do not confuse it with the Wilcoxon rank-sum test – this is a different test altogether and is equivalent to the Mann-Whitney U-test (see below).

Mann-Whitney U-test
This test is used to look for differences between two independent groups on a continuous measure (e.g. do males and females differ in terms of their self-esteem?). It requires two variables (male/female gender) and one continuous variable (self-esteem) and compares

medians. It then converts the scores on the continuous variable to ranks, where a rank is a place in a scale (see chapter 8), across the two groups. It then evaluates whether the medians for the two groups differ significantly.

Spearman rank correlation test
This test is used to demonstrate the relationship between two ranked variables. It is frequently used to compare judgements on two objects, or the scores of a group of subjects on two measures.

This is a coefficient correlation based on ranks.

The degree of relationship between two or more variables, or between two or more sets of data, is called linear correlation. The degree of relationship is expressed by the coefficient of correlation and is symbolised by r. The closer r is to 1.00 (either negative or positive) the stronger the relationship.

This test shows the association between two variables (X and Y), which are not normally distributed.

This has been no more than a brief look at some of the more common statistical tests for the analysis of data obtained from quantitative research. There are many others, and any good statistics book will detail them.

Now all these statistical tests may seem quite daunting, but if you are involved in quantitative research and have to do statistical analysis, don't worry because help is at hand. There are several computer packages that can undertake statistical analysis, for example, SPSS (**S**tatistical **P**ackage for **S**ocial **S**ciences). These programs can do just about any calculation, using any statistical test. However, you do need to know what data to enter and how to enter them, otherwise your whole research will be invalid. So, unless you have had training in the use of SPSS and similar statistical programs, you should seek the advice and help of a statistician – or at least someone who is experienced and has been trained in their use. As Botti & Endacott (2005: 192: 193) state: 'consultation with a statistician during the design phase of the research will help ensure that both the design of the study and the way data are collected enables the use of more powerful statistical analysis.'

Before we conclude this section, remember: *you need to be careful when you are looking at research that uses statistics.*

Limitations of research study/data/statistical tests

When reading research papers, always look for the section on the limitations of the methodology – the researchers should reflect on their study and discuss anything that did not make it perfect, for example:

- size of sample;
- tests used;
- initial question.

And finally ...

It is easy to get bogged down when doing statistics as part of your research or when reading research papers. You need to bear in mind four things:

1. Keep it simple.
2. Statistics in themselves are meaningless; it is their analysis and the discussion of them that make them meaningful and bring them to life.
3. 'Careful and explicit design of research investigations is required to meet the objectives of replicability, objectivity and measurement underpinning quantitative research' (Botti & Endacott 2005: 193).
4. Get to know a friendly statistician.

Scenario 1

We asked you to save the results from scenario 2 in chapter 8. Now we want you to analyse those results.

You can start by ranking each of the statements in terms of the degree to which your colleagues agree/disagree with the statement, e.g. how many strongly agree with each statement, how many agree with each statement, and so on.

Next find the arithmetic mean, the mode and the median of each of the statements (how many strongly agreed with statement 1, statement 2, and so on).

Now write an analysis of your results and what they mean for the recruitment of healthcare professionals in the future.

Keep your statistics because they will be needed for a scenario in chapter 10 – communicating research findings.

Qualitative data analysis

Introduction

We now turn to the analysis of data from qualitative research studies.

Once we have obtained the data from our qualitative research study, we need to analyse them in order to make sense of them and make accessible to the researcher (and anybody who reads a report of the research) the large amount of rich textual data that have been generated by means of the qualitative research study.

Data analysis consists of examining, categorising, tabulating and recombining the evidence obtained from the research. All this is concerned with the organisation and interpretation of information (other than numerical information, which is generally the preserve of quantitative research) in order to discover any important underlying patterns and trends.

Method of analysis

As an overview of how to analyse phenomenological research, we shall look at a method of analysis described by Kleiman (2004). Similar processes occur in other types of qualitative research.

- First you need to read the interview transcript in full in order to get an overall sense of the whole.
- You then need to read the interview transcript again – this time more slowly – in order to divide the data into meaningful sections or units. These meaningful units arise from the words of the participants.
- Following this second reading and identification of the meaningful units, you must integrate those you have identified as having a similar focus or content in order to clarify and make sense of them.
- The next stage in your analysis of the raw data (i.e. the text of the transcript) occurs with your integrated meaningful units being subjected to a process that is known as free imaginative variation. This determines which of them is essential for, and is made up of, a fixed identity for the phenomena that you are studying.
- You then need to elaborate on your findings. This includes descriptions of the essential meanings that were discovered through the process mentioned above.
- The structure of the phenomena is the major finding of any descriptive phenomenological inquiry. This structure is based on the essential meanings that are present in the descriptions of the participants and is determined by the analysis as above and by insights which arose from the process analysis to which you subjected the text.
- In the next stage, you need to look at the raw data descriptions again in order to justify the articulations of both the essential meanings and the general structure. It is of the utmost importance that you can substantiate the accuracy of all your findings from the raw data.
- Finally, once the phenomenological analysis of the data is complete, you must follow this with a critical analysis of your work within this research study. This will include verification that:
  - concrete, detailed descriptions have been obtained from the participants;
  - the phenomenological reduction has been maintained throughout the analysis;
  - essential meanings have been discovered;

- a structure has been articulated;
- the raw data have verified the results

(Kleiman 2004).

The constant comparative method

The constant comparative method is the process that is used in qualitative research by which any newly collected data are compared with previous data that were collected in one or more earlier studies (or even the same study). This is an ongoing procedure, because theories are formed, enhanced, confirmed or even discounted as a result of new data that emerge from the study.

One way in which data can be constantly compared throughout a research study is by means of coding.

Coding

Coding is the process of going through the data with a fine-tooth comb looking for themes, ideas and categories and then noting similar parts of the text and giving them a code label. This means that, at a later date, we can find them again in order to make a comparison between passages in the text and to start to analyse what is going on. Coding the data makes them easier to manage and to be able to retrieve relevant data when needed. Subsequently, we can make comparisons between categories and ideas and then identify any patterns that are worthy of further investigation as we refine concepts and themes that emerge from the text.

The codes that we use are normally based on intrinsic and extrinsic tangibles and intangibles that we identify as being relevant to our study. For example, they can be based on:

- ideas;
- concepts;
- terms;
- phrases;
- keywords.

We hope that these will lead us to a series of themes and topics so that we can start to make sense of the very rich data we are analysing and so start to understand the phenomena that are being experienced. or have been experienced, by the participants in the research study.

Although the data that we code usually arise from sections of text that we have transcribed from interviews, they may also be excerpts from diaries, audio or video recordings or even images (e.g. children's drawings). These different media are coded in the same way so that there is consistency of coding within any particular qualitative research study.

As you work through the data (whether from transcribed texts, diaries, audio or video recordings, images), the number of codes will evolve and grow as more topics or themes are identified. If a theme is identified from the data that does not quite fit the codes that you have already identified, then you have to create a new code to incorporate that theme in your analysis and interpretation.

Three types of coding are used in qualitative research:

1. **Open coding** – this is the first organisation of the data to try to make some sense of them.
2. **Axial coding** – this is a way of interconnecting the categories.
3. **Selective coding** – the building up of a story that connects the categories.

At the end of these processes, it is hoped that you will have a set of theoretical propositions (i.e. a theory to explain both the data and what is actually happening).

Now we shall look at these three types of coding in more detail.

Open coding

In open coding, the data that have been collected are divided into segments and then scrutinised for commonalities that may reflect categories or themes. Once the data have been categorised, they are examined for properties that characterise each category. (Properties are either specific attributes of a category, or they may be subcategories.)

Open coding is the process of taking the raw data and:

*   breaking them down;
*   examining them;
*   labelling them;
*   comparing them;
*   conceptualising them; and
*   categorising them.

The researcher will examine and identify the meaning of the data by:

*   identifying the meaning of the data;
*   asking questions;
*   making comparisons;
*   looking for similarities and differences between the comments.

In this way, similar comments (or incidents and events, i.e. phenomena) are grouped together to form categories.

So basically, open coding is a process of reducing the data to a small set of themes that appear to describe the phenomenon under investigation.

Axial coding

During the process of axial coding, connections are made among and between the categories and subcategories. Basically, this involves putting data together in new ways by looking for and making connections between the categories. Here the focus is on determining more about each category in terms of exploring:

- the conditions that give rise to it;
- the context in which it is embedded;
- the strategies used to manage it or to carry it out;
- the consequences of those strategies.

All of these influence the phenomena and/or social processes that are being studied. Then, as more data are collected, the researcher moves backwards and forwards among the data collection, all the time open coding and axial coding them, and continually refining the categories and their interconnections.

Selective coding

This is the process of selecting the core (or main) category and then systematically relating it to the other categories. It involves the validation of these relationships and then filling in any categories that may require further refining and/or developing.

Selective coding is the process of:

- selecting the core category;
- systematically relating it to the other categories;
- validating those relationships;
- filling in categories that require further refinement and development.

During this process, the categories and their interrelationships are combined to form a 'story-line' (or narrative) that describes what happens in the phenomenon that is being studied.

Content analysis

Another method of analysing qualitative data is by a process known as content analysis. Cavanagh (1997) notes that this method allows for the testing of theoretical issues, which in turn enhance our understanding of the data that have been engendered by the research study. According to Weber (1985), there are no universal rules of how content analysis should be used, but Downe-Wamboldt (1992) and Weber (1995) have both discussed a specific process for the conduct of content analysis. They suggest that a process could be:

1. The selection of the unit of analysis – deciding what to analyse and in what detail.

2. The creation and definition of categories – the provision of a means of describing the phenomena being studied, in order to both increase an understanding of the phenomena and to generate new knowledge.
3. The pre-testing of the definition of the category and of the rules – trial coding a sample of text in order to identify problems that may arise with the coding, or help to gain a better insight into the data.
4. The assessment of reliability – this is in terms of the reliability and stability of the data and of the particular system of coding being used.
5. The assessment of validity – does the instrument of data collection and analysis measure what it purports to measure? In this case, are the classification system, variables that have been engendered and identified, and the interpretation of data valid?
6. The revision of the rules of coding – this step is only necessary if the reliability measures are deemed to be unsatisfactory. In this case, the coding scheme needs to be revised before reassessing the reliability of the data and coding system.
7. The pre-testing of the revised category scheme – to ensure reliability and validity.
8. The coding of all the data –   all the text is coded, as are any other data that are being analysed by this method (e.g. drawings).
9. The final reassessment of reliability and validity – this is the end of the process when all the complete data are subjected to content analysis to ensure adequate reliability and validity

(Cavanagh 1997).

The coding of the data precedes their analysis, so once the data have been coded and you are satisfied that they are reliable and valid, you can start to analyse/interpret them.

Numerous – mainly numerical – strategies have been used to analyse the data (Cavanagh 1997), including:

- The use of frequency counts to compare data (Smith et al. 1983, Miller et al. 1989, Kovach et al. 1991).
- The use of category ranking (Powers et al. 1983).
- Multivariate analysis of variance (MANOVA) and multiple regression methods (Holcomb et al. 1993).

Grounded theory – analysis of data

You will recall that in grounded theory the theory develops from the data as they are collected and analysed, therefore analysis commences whilst the data collection is still taking place – the analysis may even begin when only one interview has occurred (as long as enough data have been collected at this point). One justification for doing this is that the results from the first interview can influence the direction of further interviews. Consequently, once sufficient data have been collected and transcribed, it is possible – indeed necessary – that you implement the next stage, namely compiling an indexing system for the data (Smith & Biley 1997).

The preliminary coding consists of indexing from the text following an exploration of topics or aspects that are considered to be important or interesting. These are then labelled according to their possible relevance to the topic under exploration. The aim is to build up a list of relevant topics that have emerged from the interview and are considered essential to the subject under investigation. These indexes are constructed following a line-by-line, or word-by-word, analysis of the text. It is time-consuming and demanding, but necessary to continually answer questions about what you are reading, such as 'what is important here?', 'what does this mean?', 'what is the subtext?' (Smith & Biley 1997).

Slowly a series of categories, concepts or codes are built up which start to explain the phenomena you are encountering. This process continues with all the data as they are collected, each time adding, amalgamating or even removing codes and concepts, as new data cause you to rethink what you have discovered, and possibly to change it. It is very much a dynamic process.

Following the constant comparison analysis method discussed above, the coded concepts identified in the preliminary coding analysis are now refined, extended and cross-referenced (Smith & Biley 1997). This takes place over three processes:

1. Index system refining.
2. Memorandum writing – the noting and writing of theoretical memos recording your thoughts on the nature of the phenomena, relationships among categories, codes and existing theoretical models. This should be done as soon as you think of them or you may forget them, and so lose the thread of your theory development.
3. Integration of emerging categories – searching for relationships between categories.

The end-product of all this analysis is normally the production of 'completely saturated fundamental core categories, in addition to a list of definitions, large quantities of theoretical memos, possibly linkage suggestions and a model (or number of models) that describe and explain the data' (Smith & Biley 1997: 24).

Example of analysis of text

We have discussed textual analysis, and below we give an example. This is part of an actual interview with a person who has cancer and who is talking about the support he gets from members of the palliative care team in his area.

'... the district nurse, they're only round the corner, you know. I know they're pushed, but sometimes they ... they phone me up the day before, and they're, you know, are you alright, do you need us round tomorrow, like, or what, like you know. I say, no that's alright, you can leave me out this week and come next week, whatever. I know they're there if I need them, like, and when I ... I think that's the main thing – knowing there's somebody there, you know. The district nurses, the Macmillan people, and the hospice, like you know, hospice care – just 'cos you're there on a Tuesday they don't forget about you when you leave, like you know. You can phone them up any time, like you know. It's good care, I think, I'm getting like, you know, good care.'

Now here is the same text, but this time it has been analysed for important ideas and concepts. You will see that is reproduced with the lines further apart than in the version above. This allows for the researcher's comments to be inserted within the text. This is the first stage of analysis – open coding.

Example of analysis of text

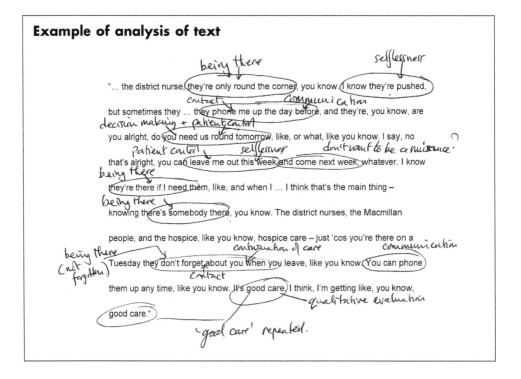

As you can see, the text has been read carefully and key terms, concepts and ideas that are considered important to the interviewee are circled and little notes are made alongside the key terms.

The second stage of the analysis of this small piece of text is to put the notes in some sort of order by combining/integrating them, looking for commonalities.

Six terms should start to emerge:

1. being there;
2. selflessness;
3. patient control;
4. communication;
5. continuation of care;
6. evaluation of care.

Now we can start to put some 'meat on the bones' by analysing the key terms and trying to explain them and their importance to the patient:

- Being there for the patient – he does not feel isolated and hence feels reassured and 'safe'.
- Selflessness of the patient – although very ill, he does not want to be a burden/nuisance and is thinking of others (the nurses? other patients?). Also, perhaps he wants to maintain some control over his life (see next point).
- Patient control identified by his decision-making – being able to make decisions as to what he wants and what he can do. In this way he is still retaining some control over his life, even though he is close to death. By retaining some control, he is maintaining his dignity – he is not passive and accepting, but rather is active in his life. His illness is not robbing him of that.
- Good communication and contact with members of the palliative care team – this is important to him in order to feel 'safe' and reassured and to realise that he is not facing his disease and the consequences of it alone.
- Continuation of care – the fact that he is not forgotten by members of the palliative care team between the visits is important to him as it gives him reassurance and allows him to feel 'safe'.
- Qualitative evaluation – although he cannot objectively evaluate his care, what is important to him is that he perceives that he is getting good care from the palliative care services. The fact that he repeats the phrase 'good care' in the same sentence demonstrates its importance to him.

You can see that even a short excerpt like this one can give you a lot of detail for analysis.

From this extract and the notes made alongside it, you can take it further and see similarities between some of the points above, and that some themes can emerge as bigger than the individual notes and points, for example, 'control' is very important to this patient and appears in several of the points above under different guises. Other themes to appear are 'reassurance' and 'safety'

Thus, from this one short excerpt, we can start to get to know the interviewee and to understand his concerns and feelings. In particular, we start to understand the story he is telling of how he is living with a phenomenon that is novel to him – living with cancer.

This is not the whole of his story though – it is but a brief extract. As we textually analyse the whole of the interview and marry this to field notes taken at the time of the interview, we can start to construct a broader picture of what he is telling us.

Scenario

In chapter 8, we asked you to record the interview in which you were the interviewee and a friend the interviewer. Now we want you to transcribe that interview (if you are short of time, transcribe just one or two pages of it).

The next stage is to analyse the full or partial transcript as we have done in the example above. Do any themes emerge? If so write them down, and then write a short report on the results of your analysis. The more you practise this, the better at identifying concepts and themes you will become.

Keep your transcript, because you will need it for a scenario in chapter 10 – communicating research findings.

Analysis of images

'According to Oster and Gould (1987), human figure drawings can be used as projective instruments which can be analysed for emotional indicators. The emphasis on the drawings can then be centred on the child's emotional conflict and attitudes rather than just on the milestones of development' (Vickers 2009: 287–288).

These can be grouped into three categories:

1. Overall quality of the figure, including the line quality, proportions and shading.
2. Untypical specific features, such as a large or small head, accentuated teeth, crossed eyes.
3. The inclusion of typical features, including the eyes, nose, feet and neck.

However, for some children, drawing a human figure can be perceived as threatening in certain scenarios, so in order to produce more useful information from this approach, alternatives are now used. The children are asked to draw houses and trees (among other objects and situations), the assumption being that each drawing will tap into various segments of the child's personality. For example, a house is thought to link with issues of family ties as well as with conflicts surrounding home life. This link is also identified with family drawings in which importance is given to the child's perceived position within the family hierarchy. For example, if children feel important, they will usually place themselves next to their parent(s). Children who feel isolated or 'different' may place themselves in the margin of the picture, or even draw themselves as physically separated from other members of their family (e.g. by a line or by a table),

In Figure 9.1, an eight-year-old boy sees himself as the link that holds the family together (his parents were experiencing relationship difficulties at the time), so rather than using lines to separate him from his parents, he uses the lines to maintain a connection with them both and so allows his parents to remain connected to each other.

This is just one example of the way in which drawings can form part of your data so that topics and themes can emerge from the analysis, just as they do from written text. The analysis of non-verbal data is more specialised than is the analysis of verbal/written data, but it can

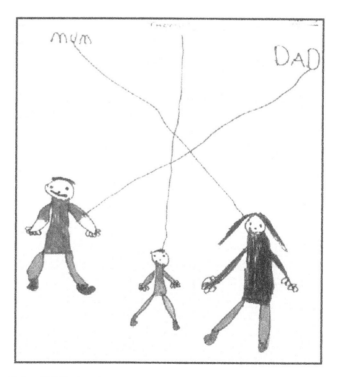

Figure 9.1 Child's drawing
Reproduced with permission from Vickers P. S. (2009) *Severe combined immune deficiency: Early hospitalisation and isolation.* Chichester: Wiley-Blackwell

provide insights that you might not be able to obtain from other forms of data, particularly when working with young children.

Summary of qualitative data analysis

Qualitative data analysis is the process in which we move from the raw qualitative data that have been collected during the research study and use it to attempt to provide explanations, understanding and interpretation of the phenomena, people and situations we are studying. The aim of analysing qualitative data is to examine the meaningful and symbolic content of people's/groups' experiences and of events that occur in their lives – cultural, social, psychological and individual.

What we are aiming for is the identification and an understanding of such concepts, situations and ideas as:

- A person's interpretation of the world/situation in which they find themselves at any given moment.
- How they have arrived at that point of view in terms of their situation or world/environment in which they find themselves.
- How they relate to others in their world.
- Practical issues (e.g. how they cope).
- Their view of their own personal history and the history of others in their social milieu.
- How they identify and see themselves and others in their own situation/environment.

Qualitative data analysis usually involves the identification and explanation of themes. Although writing of some kind is found in almost all forms of qualitative data analysis, the raw data may come from other media (e.g. images or observation). However, it is certainly a truism that discovering and identifying themes comprise much of the role of the qualitative researcher.

Summary

That concludes the brief discourse on the analysis of data obtained from the quantitative and the qualitative paradigms. It is impossible to cover, in depth or in range, all the elements of quantitative and qualitative data analysis, but there are many books and web programs on specific types of data analysis and it is important that before you decide on your method of data analysis, you become very familiar and confident in your chosen field. The advice given throughout this chapter is to seek help and advice if you are not certain of what you should be doing, and we reiterate this advice here.

The research proposal is almost completed once you have included the method of data analysis you will be using to answer your research question. You will still have a few things to sort out – for example, the dissemination of your findings (this is covered in chapter 10 as well as in the web program), and the resources (also in the web program). However, as you expand the research proposal, it is very important to keep going back to other parts of your research proposal and making changes in light of what you have learned as you have worked through these later chapters and have gained new knowledge and a deeper understanding of the process.

Activity

Ask a group of friends or colleagues for a numerical statistic – e.g. their age, height, number of children. Then rank them and perform three statistical tests – the arithmetic mean, the median and the mode. Is there any difference between these averages? Can you work out why the differences occur – are some members of your group much older or younger than the majority, or do they have many more children than the rest?

References

Black S. (1997) Quantitative studies (editorial). *Nurse Researcher* **4**(4): 3.

Botti M. & Endacott R. (2005) Clinical research 5: Quantitative data collection and analysis. *Intensive and Critical Care Nursing* **21**: 187–193.

Burns N. & Grove S. K. (2005) *The practice of nursing research: Conduct, critique, and utilization* (5th edition). St Louis, MO: Elsevier Saunders.

Carlyle T. (1840) *Chartism*. London: James Fraser.

Cavanagh S. (1997) Content analysis: concepts, methods and applications. *Nurse Researcher* **4**(3): 5–16.

Crookes P. A. & Davies S. (Eds.) (2004) *Research into practice: Essential skills for reading and applying research in nursing and health care* (2nd edition). Edinburgh: Baillière Tindall.

Disraeli B. (1804–1881) attributed and quoted in A. B. Paine (Ed.) (1924) *Mark Twain's Autobiography* (p. 246). London: Harper Brothers.

Downe-Wamboldt B. (1992) Content analysis: method, applications and issues. *Health Care for Women International* **13**(3): 313–321.

Hinton P. R. (1995) *Statistics explained: A guide for social science students*. London: Routledge.

Holcomb L. E., Neimeyer R. A. & Moore M. K. (1993). Personal meanings of death: A content analysis of free-response narratives. *Death Studies* **17**: 299–318.

Kleiman S. (2004) Phenomenology: to wonder and search for meanings. *Nurse Researcher* **11**(4): 7–19.

Koosis D. J. (1997) *Statistics: A self-teaching guide*. Chichester: John Wiley & Sons.

Kovach C. R. (1991) Content analysis of reminiscences of elderly women. *Research in Nursing and Health* **14**: 287–295.

Miller P., McMahon M., Garrett M. J. & Ringel K. (1989) A content analysis of life adjustments post-infarction. *Western Journal of Nursing Research* **11**: 559–567.

Neutens J. J. & Rubinson L. (2002) *Research techniques for the health sciences* (3rd edition). San Francisco: Benjamin Cummings.

Pallant J. (2001) *SPSS survival manual: A step by step guide to data analysis using SPSS*. Buckingham: Open University Press.

Powers M. J., Murphy S. P. & Wooldridge P. J. (1883) Validation of two experimental nursing approaches using content analysis. *Research in Nursing & Health* **6**(**1**): 3–9.

Oster G. D. & Gould P. (1987) *Using drawings in assessment and theory: A guide for mental health professionals*. New York: Brunner/Mazell

Shorter Oxford English Dictionary (6th edition 2007). Oxford: Oxford University Press.

Sim J. & Wright C. (2000) *Research in health care: Concepts, designs and methods*. London: Stanley Thornes

Smith C. E., Garvis M. S. & Martinson I. M. (1983) Content analysis of interviews using a nursing model: A look at parents adapting to the impact of childhood cancer. *Cancer Nursing* **6**(**4**): 269–275.

Smith K. & Biley F. (1997) Understanding grounded theory: principles and evaluation. *Nurse Researcher* **4**(**3**): 17–30.

Vickers P. S. (2009) *Severe combined immune deficiency: Early hospitalisation and isolation*. Chichester: Wiley-Blackwell.

Weber R. P. (1985) *Basic content analysis*. Newbury Park, CA: Sage.

Weber R. P. (1995) Basic content analysis. In M. S. Lewis-Beck (Ed.) *Research practice. International handbooks of quantitative application in the social sciences* (Vol. 6). London: Sage.

The Research Proposal: Communicating Research Findings

Introduction

This chapter is linked to the dissemination of findings section of the web program. Unlike the previous chapters in this book, it is not devoted to the theory behind the research in order to provide you with the tools to help you to write a research proposal. Rather, it gives you practical tips to help you with:

- writing your research report;
- writing for publication;
- presenting at a conference.

These are all important aspects of your research study and as you must disseminate your results in order to validate your research, we have included practical advice on how to do this.

You may have thought that your research proposal was complete. However, you would be wrong. You may have included in your research proposal the collection and analysis of your data, but even when you have done that, your study is far from over. It is only completed when you have written your research report and disseminated the findings (you need to mention this in your research proposal) and possibly implemented them (see chapter 11 and the web program).

Once you have written your report, you still have to communicate your findings to your colleagues, peers and others interested in your subject. This chapter gives you some tips on how to write a research report at the end of the study, and then explains how you can go about disseminating your research study, especially its findings and recommendations, to as wide an audience as possible. There are two main ways of doing this:

1. writing for publication;
2. presentations at conferences.

However, before we look at these, there are some other people who need to be apprised of your findings. These are the people who participated in your research as subjects and without whose participation your research would not have taken place. Do not overlook them. You need to have in place some means of letting them know the results of their endeavours on your behalf. Some of the ways in which this can be done are:

- Letting them see copies of the final research report – perhaps by making it available in the hospital or clinic.
- Giving each of them a copy of the executive summary.
- Meeting them individually to discuss your results and recommendations, and possibly implementation.
- Meeting them in groups to disseminate the results and recommendations.
- Telephoning them.

Finally, do not forget to send them a note of thanks (this should be included in your research proposal, as the research ethics committee in particular will expect this).

The following sections are concerned with the dissemination of your results to colleagues and peers and mainly offer practical advice on what to do and what not to do. We begin with writing the final research report and then look at writing papers for publication.

Writing a research report

The plan of your research report is similar to your proposal, with the exception that your proposal is written in the future tense whilst the report is written in the past tense (Munhall & Chenail 2008).

The other major differences are that the research proposal does not contain sections on results and discussion, as well as recommendations, whilst the research report will need these in order to be complete.

The box is a plan for a quantitative research study.

Plan of a research report for a quantitative study into pain relief

- Contents
- Acknowledgements
- Executive summary

Part One: Introduction
- Introduction – including background to the research and aims of the study
- Review of literature
- Research methodology

Part Two: Research findings
- Results – introduction
- Results – statistics

Part Three: Discussion and conclusion
- Discussion
- Conclusion and recommendations

Part Four: References
- References
Appendices

Next is an example of the plan of a research proposal for a recent study into palliative care. The plan for the subsequent research report following the completion of the study appears in the third box.

If you work through the linked web program on writing a research proposal, you will see this proposal in full. In this chapter, only the headings are given.

Plan of a research proposal for a qualitative study into palliative care

- Title
- Abstract – summary
- Introduction – purpose of the research (Aim)
- Background and literature review
- Outcomes
- Study design – Methodology
- Subjects:
  - inclusion/exclusion criteria
  - method of recruitment
  - potential problems
- The health and comfort of the subjects
- Ethical considerations
- Resources
- References

Plan of a research report for a qualitative study into palliative care

- Contents
- Acknowledgements
- Executive summary

Part One: Introduction
- Introduction – including background to the research and aims of the study
- Review of literature
- Research methodology

Part Two: Research findings
- Results – introduction
- Results – patients
- Results – carers and families
- Results – palliative care team members

Part Three: Discussion and conclusion
- Discussion
- Conclusion and recommendations

Part Four: References
- References
Appendices

This was a phenomenological qualitative research study looking at the perceptions of adults with cancer accessing palliative care services, their families and members of the palliative care teams in the area, regarding the needs of the patients and families, and whether the palliative care services were meeting those needs.

Another significant difference between a research proposal and a research report is their length. For example, for this study, the proposal is three pages long and the research report is 270 pages long, excluding the appendices, which themselves total 60 pages.

Research reports

Concentrating for now on the research reports, you can see from the two examples that the sections within the plans are very similar for both the quantitative and qualitative research studies; the major differences between them lie in the research findings sections, with the quantitative research study being concerned with the presentation and analysis of statistics, whilst the qualitative research study is concerned with the presentation and analysis of the text from interviews and focus groups.

So, let us look at the research reports in more detail.

Contents

This is simply a list of the chapters and sections in your report and the page numbers so that a reader can easily locate any chapter or section. For example:

Chapter Three: Research methodology		
Subsection	**Contents**	**Page**
3.1	Introduction	48
3.2	Qualitative methodology	50
3.3	Sample	57
And so on.		

Acknowledgements

This comes at the beginning of your report where you acknowledge the people who have helped with your research – particularly the participants. Others usually acknowledged are colleagues and people who have helped in any way.

Executive summary

This is a summary of your research which, although part of your research, can be detached and given to people who do not want to read the whole report. It usually includes the title of the study, the background to the study, the aim/hypothesis and objectives, a brief note on the methodology and, most importantly, the key findings and recommendations. This is also usually signed by the researcher(s). It can also be printed as a separate document because many of the users will be happy just to have the results, which should be given prominence in the executive summary.

Introduction

This includes the background to the study (in more detail than is found in the executive summary) and the aims/hypothesis of the study. A review of literature linked to the topic of the study is included, as is the methodology (much of this can be taken from the research proposal – although do remember to change the tenses of the verbs from the future to the past).

Research findings

This is usually a straightforward account and analysis of the findings from the study. It may be in the form of statistics or of whatever data you collected from a qualitative study. The statistical tests and the statistics themselves often follow on one from another, although they may be grouped in related sets. Qualitative data are often presented within the themes that you have identified from the data.

Discussion
This is the section where you discuss the results and try to make sense of them in the context of your research study. This is the crux of your report because it can include the conclusions from the report, recommendations arising from the data and analysis of data, and implications for practice. Reflections on the study – the way you carried it out, any problems or weaknesses (and strengths) with your research study and suggestions for further research that have arisen also come in this section.

References
As with any academic work, this is where you include the references you have cited in the text of your report. These references mainly appear in the introduction, review of literature, research methodology and discussion sections, although some may be found in the results section – but these are few, if they occur there at all. Remember to ensure that your references are given accurately and in full, and that none is missing.

Appendices
This is where you add (append) any important documents related to the research which you do not think are appropriate to include in the main body of the report (e.g. information sheets about the study, interview guides).

Summary
You can see that the first few sections can remain almost as they were in your research proposal, except for changes or alterations that needed to take place during the study itself (Munhall & Chenail 2008).

You can see now that the research proposal leads eventually to the research report, so it is very important that your proposal is as full and complete as possible – this will make it easy for you to write your final report. In the same way, if you write your report fully and accurately, and include a very good, comprehensive, but succinct, executive summary, this will help you when you come to disseminate your findings. You will be able to use sections of your report for publication or for presentations without having to change things too much.

This leads on to the next two sections – writing for publication and presenting at conferences.

Writing for publication

Writing for publication is a worthwhile endeavour – indeed, for some healthcare professionals it is essential, as it forms part of their employment contract. However, writing for publication does not come naturally to everyone. To be successful, the twin attributes of practice and perseverance are important.

Before you commence writing, there are a few points to consider. These include the type of writing that you wish to pursue and could be:

- a research paper (also referred to as an article or a manuscript);
- a book;
- a report;
- a short article.

In this section we focus on issues pertaining to writing a research article for a peer- reviewed journal. The discussion is divided into three sections:

- getting started;
- developing a detailed structure of your work;
- issues associated with healthcare professionals and publication.

Getting started

Among the first things to do is to decide on the area in which you are interested and the line you wish to take – what aspect of the topic you want to write about and for whom exactly it is intended.

Albert (2009) suggests developing a broad plan of what you intend to write about, so, using landscape orientation (i.e. the longer measure being used as the width) A4 paper (or larger), draw a large circle in the middle of the sheet. Write the theme of your topic in the centre of the circle. Working outwards from this circle, draw lines to connect four smaller circles, two on each side of the larger circle. In each of the small circles, write:

- Why did we start?
- What did we do?
- What did we find?
- What does it mean?

To answer these questions, use lines and arrows to make connections with items or points in your paper. This is known as 'mind mapping' (Buzan 1993). Continue until you believe that you have enough information to formulate major headings for your paper. At this preliminary stage, you may wish to discuss your ideas with colleagues.

During this start-up period, you should set yourself feasible goals and stick to them.

Murray & Moore (2006) advocate viewing the writing of your article as a project which should have specific activities, accompanied by instructions to yourself for each of the activities.

Decide on your audience and journal

You should think carefully about your target audience and choose a suitable peer-reviewed journal that you know is read by them. A peer-reviewed (or refereed) journal is one which subjects all articles that are submitted to it for publication to critical assessment by independent scholars working in the same area as the author before it is even considered for acceptance for publication. A common practice is for an article to be double-blind peer-reviewed. This means that the names of the author and the reviewers are not revealed to each other. The reviewers recommend whether the article should be accepted, revised or rejected based on specific criteria set by the journal. The process is the accepted method for ensuing fairness, high quality information and contribution of new knowledge to the field. However, do be aware that some articles which appear in peer-reviewed journals may not have undergone peer review; these include book reviews, news items and editorials. However, basically anything that you submit will be peer-reviewed.

Peer-reviewed journals have *Instructions for Authors*. These are the house style of how articles should be written and are sometimes found in the journal, but are certainly found on the journal's webpage. It is important that you familiarise yourself with these instructions and also with the layout of articles which appear in your selected journal and adapt your work accordingly so that it fits in with the journal's house style, for example:

- Presentation style: do they use 'Introduction' or 'Background'? Are there any limitations on the number of tables, figures or references? What are the font requirements?
- What referencing style do they use? Do they have a particular variation on the style?
- What types of articles are accepted – research-based, evaluation or service development?
- Familiarise yourself with the submission details – e.g. length, turnaround time.
- Your covering letter to the editor(s) should 'sell' your article – but note, you do not usually get paid; the prestige of being published is supposed to be sufficient reward. Also make sure that you send your article to one journal at a time – do **not** mass mail it to all the journals you can think of, because the journals do communicate with each other and will discard any article that has been sent to another journal.

You may also wish to check the journal's rating. This is particularly important for academic research writers as some journals are more highly rated than others and publications in these journals have relevance for the assessment of research quality in all higher education institutions in the UK. The higher education funding bodies use the quality profiles to determine the grant for research to the institutions (http://www.rae.ac.uk and http://www.hefce.ac.uk/research/ref/).

Review the literature

You should provide up-to-date literature about your topic (see chapter 4). You should also be able to articulate how your current work supports/refutes what is already available. Your literature review should contain a critique of the papers under discussion and the contribution your work will make to the debate.

Draft an outline of your work

An early draft of your work helps with the structure of the paper (Albert 2009). Murray (2006: 195) employs Brown's eight questions strategy to focus writing:

1.   Who are the intended readers? (3–5 names)
2.   What did I do? (50 words answering this question)
3.   Why did I do it? (50 words)
4.   What happened? (50 words)
5.   What do the results mean in theory? (50 words)
6.   What do the results mean in practice? (50 words)
7.   What is the key benefit for readers? (25 words)
8.   What remains unresolved? (no word limit)

These questions are designed to be used as a tool for outlining the paper and provide a device for checking the coherence of your work.

Comments from colleagues

This is a useful procedure to undertake as constructive critical comments may broaden your outlook of the topic or provide another way of expressing your ideas.

Develop a detailed structure for the paper

The basic structure of research paper is formatted sequentially, as follows:

• Introduction
• Methods
• Results

and

• Discussion

This is usually referred to as IMRaD.

An overview (Gray 2004, Parahoo 2006, Houser 2008, Polit & Beck 2008) of each of these is explained below. However, you must bear in mind the journal's requirements as each journal will differ in the detail of what they expect, particularly their word limit for articles.

The abstract

This is usually written last as it contains an extract from your paper. It provides the reader with a summary of the contents of your paper. Typically an abstract includes:

- an outline of the background and the objective of the paper;
- the principal activity of the study and its scope;
- minimal information about the methodology;
- the most important results emerging from the study;
- a statement of conclusion or recommendation.

The abstract should 'sell' your work and entice the reader to read the entire paper. It really is worthwhile spending a lot of time writing a good abstract, because in many instances this is the only part of the paper that gets read! (See also chapter 4.)

Reflect on the literature search you carried out for your own topic – you may only have been able to read the abstract because some abstracts are published in abstract journals or online databases. This highlights the need to provide the essential features of your work in your own abstract.

Some journals ask you to provide keywords which, when accepted, are stored electronically along with titles and abstracts. This is very useful, because you probably remember using keywords, which you typed in the database, for the literature search you undertook for your topic and this was followed by a printout of titles of articles appearing on the computer screen containing those keywords (which are often highlighted). So you can see that it is vital that your keywords reflect what your paper contains so that others can retrieve information from it and subsequently retrieve your paper for reading.

Introduction

This section should contain:

- the background to the area under discussion;
- a critical discussion of the literature;
- identification of the research problem;
- an explanation of the theoretical/conceptual framework (if appropriate);
- the aims and objectives/hypothesis of study.

Methods

Your methods section should include:

- an explanation and justification of the research paradigm that you used;
- the rationale for your sampling approach, a description of the study setting and how you selected the participants;
- a justification of your data collection strategies;

- the identification of the main study variables;
- a description of the intervention that you use (if applicable);
- all ethical considerations related to your research study;
- a discussion of the issues that relate to the validity and reliability of your study (if applicable);
- a discussion of the issues that relate to the trustworthiness and rigour of the study (if applicable);
- a justification of the data analysis techniques that you employed.

Results
This section should include all the relevant points in this list:

- a clear and coherent presentation of all the relevant data;
- a report on response rates (if applicable);
- all numerical data presented in tables, figures and other graphical representation must be clearly and adequately labelled (if applicable);
- all verbal data clearly and simply described and accurately interpreted (if applicable);
- strict anonymity of participants;
- a description of the participants (making sure that you maintain their anonymity);
- interpretation of the results that are consistent with the results.

Discussion
The discussion section allows you the freedom to interpret the study. It should examine critically:

- key findings of the research in relation to the research questions and the literature discussed in the review and any literature subsequently found to be relevant, analysing similarities and differences between your findings and those in the literature;
- methodological issues, including strengths, limitations and issues relating to rigour.

Conclusions
These will cover:

- the extent to which the research aims and objectives have been addressed;
- the implications, significance and recommendations of the study for professional practice, management or education;
- suggestions for further research.

Acknowledgements
This section is reserved for those whom you may wish to thank for their support, for example, funding bodies, sponsors, participants in the research or critical readers who guided you during the writing process.

References
All references must accord to the journal's house style.

Issues associated with healthcare professionals and publication

There is an increasing expectation that healthcare professionals will disseminate their work and so contribute to improving practice and patient care, as well as forming an increasingly important part of their professional development. Nelms (2004) considers that writing for publication is essential to the advancement of the nursing profession (and other healthcare professionals), whilst Paul (2002) sees that a body of researched and evidence-based knowledge is the key to a developing academic profession.

However, writing for publication is a skill and requires time. Unfortunately, many healthcare professionals may not have these qualities or may not have had any formal training in academic writing (Murray & Moore 2006). Other barriers to writing include:

- lack of confidence in their skills and in their research;
- fear of rejection – by the journal initially, but also by peers, who may be critical of their paper once it is published;
- a lack of understanding about the writing process and procedures;
- too many other commitments.

However, writing and getting a paper published is a rewarding exercise. Service redesign as a result of government policy (Department of Health 2006a, 2006b, 2008) offers opportunities for healthcare professionals to communicate and disseminate new ways of working (Offredy et al. 2008), which may then be used to revise and improve patient care.

Publication has other advantages, such as informing clinical intervention and assisting in the journey to ensure that healthcare theory is applied to practice, so further increasing the research and evidence base of clinical and academic practice (Clarke 2000).

Nonetheless, you should be aware of some of the pitfalls of submitting typescripts which result in rejection (Perneger & Hudelson 2004, Morse 2007), many of which are avoidable. These are summarised in Table 10.1.

It should be noted that the reasons for accepting a typescript do not mirror the reasons for rejecting them. Morse (2007: 1164) sums up acceptance of an article in one word: that they are 'strong'. She explains that this means that:

- The article is balanced.
- The article uses adequate quotations to illustrate or convince of the rigour of the paper.

Table 10.1 Reasons for rejection of submitted typescripts.

- The paper does not contribute any new thinking to the literature.
- Inaccurate, incomplete or outdated literature.
- The research question is not specified.
- There is an imbalance in the amount of information presented in each of the sections of the paper.
- The structure of the paper is incoherent (e.g. methods are described in the Results section).
- Inadequate or insufficient description/discussion of methods, instruments and intervention.
- Results do not relate to the main research question.
- The paper does not follow the journal's instructions to authors.
- The paper exceeds the journal's word limit.
- Key arguments are unsupported by appropriate references.
- Quotations have not been attributed.
- The discussion does not answer the research question.
- The discussion and conclusions speculate beyond what has been shown in the paper.
- There are missing data (e.g. drop-outs, non-responders), for which there is no account.
- Ethical violations.
- The paper is poorly written (e.g. poor English grammar, style and syntax).
- Plagiarism (i.e. using others' work and passing it off as your own) is suspected.

(adapted from Bordage 2001, Perneger & Hudelson 2004, Morse 2007).

- The discussion explains the contribution of the research to the topic area, that is, the researchers/authors are stating their claim to knowledge.
- The article discusses the strengths and weaknesses of the study.

In other words, typescripts are accepted because of their contribution and relevance to the field to which they relate, for the excellence of the writing and for the quality of the study design and analysis (Bordage 2001).

Summary

This section has discussed a number of important points you should consider when thinking about writing for publication. It has also demonstrated that some of the common errors resulting in rejection can be avoided if attention is paid to the journal's specific requirements. The section has concluded by highlighting that the task of writing and getting published is rewarding as well as contributing to the evidence base of practice. However, in terms of your research proposal, it is enough to say, regarding publication, something along the lines of 'dissemination will be through the writing of papers for peer-reviewed journals within the sphere of the subject matter of the research study'.

Scenario 1

You have undertaken research into the reasons for people becoming healthcare professionals (refer to scenario 2 in chapter 8 and scenario 1 in chapter 9). You have the data that you collected and analysed. Now you want to write up your research for a professional journal.

However, for it to be accepted, you need to write a brief paper for the journal. Do this using the data that you have collected and analysed, using the format presented above. Try to keep your paper between 500 and 1,000 words.

This will give you some practice in writing a research paper.

Presenting at conferences

This is another important way of disseminating your research. Conferences are a regular occurrence world wide, so it is not hard to find a conference that will fit in with the topic and methodologies of your research study. However, being accepted to present your research at the conference is not always easy and can require a lot of thought and work on your part before you can even think about your presentation.

First of all, you have to know your conference:

- What is its theme?
- Does your research fit within the theme of the conference?
- What level of researcher is it aimed at – novice researcher, experienced researcher, nurse researcher, medical researcher, bioscience researcher, academic researcher – or is it aimed at healthcare professionals who are not researchers themselves, but believe that your research will help to improve their practice?
- You also have to determine where among this list of researchers and practitioners your experience and research/practice should lie.
- Where is the conference taking place?
- Can you get funding for the conference itself as well as for travelling expenses and accommodation expenses?
- Can you get the time off work to attend the conference?

If you have decided that the conference is the right one for you and that you can obtain the funding and the time to attend it, the first thing that you will have to consider and write is an abstract.

As with writing for publication, an abstract is your gateway to presenting at any conference, so as much, if not more, thought needs to go into writing your abstract as into preparing the presentation itself. Also, if accepted, your abstract may well be published in a prestigious journal, along with all the others abstracted from the conference, in which case it will be read worldwide.

Before writing the abstract, think about the theme of the conference and which part of your research fits the theme and you would like to present. You are going to have to tailor your research not only to the theme of the conference but also to the audience who will be present.

It is important to be aware that, as with writing a paper for publication, your abstract could well be rejected by the conference abstract selection committee. If this happens, don't become despondent but use it as a spur to improve your abstract for the next conference you think is suitable for you to present your research.

It may well be that your research is worth presenting, but that your abstract was not good enough or did not fit the criteria of that particular conference. Often you can get feedback from the conference abstract selection committee on why your abstract was not accepted. Or you may wish to show your abstract to a colleague experienced in submitting abstracts and presenting at conferences. However, it may be something as simple as there being so many abstracts submitted, that no matter how good yours was, there was insufficient time to include it. If that was the case, when you next decide to submit an abstract, try to ensure that it stands out from the others.

Abstract

What is an abstract? An abstract is a brief synopsis or summary of your research project. It is usually about 250 words long, and in those 250 words you have to explain:

* what the research was about;
* why you undertook that particular research;
* how you carried it out (e.g. methodology);
* what your results demonstrated and what they mean;
* why your results are significant;
* the implications for practice (if relevant).

If you look up 'abstract' in a research book or on the web, you will find a lot of helpful advice on what your abstract should contain and how you should set it out. You also need to take on board the advice given by the conference organisers because each conference, as with each journal, will have its own rules and guidelines for writing and submission of abstracts, and any failure to follow these guidelines usually means automatic disqualification. Many conference organisers will even provide a template for an abstract; this is very useful because you then know exactly what they require. For example, if you are submitting an abstract for a piece of quantitative research, your abstract may require the following headings:

- An introduction – the overall topic of the research, background to the research and reasons for undertaking this research.
- Your hypothesis or research aim.
- If applicable, your experimental approach – how did you attempt to prove/disprove your hypothesis? (There is no need to go into any detail.)
- A concise description or summary of your most important results.
- A conclusion – why your results are significant and the implications of your results for practice (if they are relevant).

On the other hand, if you are submitting a qualitative research abstract, then it may require:

- The aim of the study – the phenomenon of interest.
- The method of inquiry – this will include the type of qualitative methodology that you used (e.g. ethnographic, phenomenological), and why you used it for this particular research study.
- Your data collection instruments – which instruments you used, why you used them and how you used them.
- The findings from your study – a brief synopsis.
- Reflection and summary – a résumé of the meanings of your findings and any indications/implications for practice

(Munhall & Chenail 2008).

How does this work in practice? Remember that these two guidelines for abstracts are theoretical in order to give you some idea of the type of information that you will need to include in your abstract for it to be considered by the conference abstract committee. The crucial thing is to follow the guidelines that are given.

Below are two examples of recent successfully submitted abstracts for international conferences. When you read them, you can see that the guidelines were very different and were tailored to fit in with the guidelines.

Example of Abstract 1

The nursing care of children with severe combined immune deficiency and their families

Severe Combined Immune Deficiency (SCID) is a disorder that is rare but is fatal without successful treatment. The care of these children is a combination of curative treatment and palliative therapies to keep them alive until the treatments have worked. Whilst the nurse may well have a role to play in the actual treatment, the major role of the nurse is concerned with the palliative therapies.

The role of the nurse in the care of these children (and their families) consists of a combination of physical, psychosocial, and emotional care. Perhaps the most important role is the prevention of infections by means of very strict hygiene, observation for early signs of infections, and isolation procedures. In addition, meeting the nutritional needs of the children is a crucial role for nurses, because without good nutrition, the children are at a greater risk of succumbing to any infectious organisms that they may encounter. The dedication and concentration of the nurses in the care of the children are key to their survival until their transplant has taken. This intensive and long-term care can be very stressful for nurses, and this has to be acknowledged both by themselves and by other members of the care team.

In addition to the physical care, nurses are the major providers of psychosocial and emotional care, not only for the infants, but also for the families. Two of the major psychosocial and emotional problems that both infants and families have to face are those of isolation and separation (Vickers 2009). Other problems are linked to the developmental needs of the infants, and, of great concern, the potential for the development of Post Traumatic Stress Symptoms/Disorder (PTSS/PTSD) in children and families following a successful transplant. In addition to the risk of PTSS/PTSD, other later problems that have been noted in the children are connected with behaviour and with failing relationships.

This presentation will commence with a brief introduction and explanation of the development of treatment for children with SCID and the future treatments. It will explore the various roles, within the physical, psychosocial and emotional care, of the nurses looking after children with SCID and their families. In particular, there will be opportunities for discussions and explorations of the role of the nurse, taking into account the experiences of participants.

Reference

Vickers P. S. (2009) *Severe combined immune deficiency: Early hospitalisation and isolation.* Chichester: Wiley-Blackwell.

Example of Abstract 2

Title: Using a Virtual Learning Environment (VLE) to reach students who would not normally be able to access a course.
Presenters: *[names of the presenters are placed here]*
Aim:
To demonstrate the effectiveness of a VLE in reaching out to students wishing to study from anywhere in the world.

Abstract

Five years ago, the university decided to offer a Master's degree in immunology for health professionals, not only in the UK, but also abroad. For several reasons – including pedagogical, practical and economic – it was decided that the way forward was by means of a VLE.

Technology needs to ensure that students are fully engaged in learning (Glen, 2005) as the expectation of many students is that education will be flexible and accessible for their needs, so from the student point of view, and in line with stated Government policy (DfES 2003), the many advantages include:

- Flexibility is built into these programmes.
- Life-long learning: The student can save the web links in order to keep returning to it after the degree for regular updating.
- It can be accessed from anywhere in the world wherever there is access to the internet.

A VLE is an ideal medium for education as working in collaboration supports learning through interaction with others (Tam 2000). A VLE aids the acquisition of theory to practice, develops reflective practice and most importantly, allows the student to take responsibility for their own learning.

Some of the strengths of the VLE is that it can reach diverse groups anywhere in the world, is interactive, versatile, and flexible.

This presentation will discuss the difficulties, advantages, and practicalities of setting up and running a degree using a VLE.

Learning Outcomes

At the end of this presentation, participants will:

- Have an understanding of the value of using a VLE to deliver a module or course.
- Be able to discuss the advantages and disadvantages of using a VLE to deliver education.
- Appreciate the practicalities of developing a VLE for students locally, nationally and internationally.

Keywords

- VLE
- Flexibility
- Accessibility

References

DfES (2003) *The future of higher education*. Norwich: The Stationery Office.
Tam M. (2000) Constructivism, instructional design, and technology: Implications for transforming distance learning. *Educational Technology and Society* 3(2): 50–60.

Preparation for the conference

Let us assume that your abstract has been accepted by the conference abstract selection committee. Now you have to prepare both yourself and your material for the conference itself.

If you have never stood in front of an audience and given a presentation, the very thought of it can be exhilarating or, more likely, terrifying. How can you make sure that you are prepared for the conference? There are several things that you can do to help yourself.

- First of all, make sure that your slides are perfect. Do not try to cram too much on any slide, but just give the essential points of your presentation. Below are two examples of slides for presentations (the first one is made up – and is actually the information from three slides put on one).

Key Findings & Recommendations

- Support for bereaved family members.
- Dynamic & flexible service. –allows for individual initiatives to deal with situations as they arise and to care for varies needs.
- Willingness by individual members of the palliative care team to go that 'extra mile' to care for and help patients and families.
- Excellent working relationships between different parts of the palliative care services
- Some problems in relation to communication and co-ordination with palliative care services, e.g. General Practitioners
- Lack of support for the children of parents who have incurable cancer
- Lack of knowledge and information in the private health care system
- Education for palliative care health professionals
- Bereavement support (time span)
- Accessibility of palliative care services for those from ethnic minorities
- Concern over the Self-Directed Care scheme
- Need for peer/social support
- Bereavement support (time span)
- Accessibility of palliative care services for those from ethnic minorities
- Concern over the Self-Directed Care scheme
- Need for peer/social support

The type size here is too small, making it difficult to read. The background is 'fussy' and is not conducive to easy reading of the text. There is also too much information, so the audience could lose interest before you have finished the slide – if you have 10 such slides, then you will really 'lose' your audience, no matter how interesting the material and presentation.

"LIVING WITH CANCER"

Methods:

▹ **Interviews:**
  ◦ Individual with the patient or carer/family member
  ◦ With both patient and family member/carer
  ◦ Home environment
▹ **Focus Groups:**
  ◦ With professionals
  ◦ Professional environment

From the same presentation, this slide conveys the right amount of information – basically headings of the material discussed by the presenter. It is on a 'clean' background and the print is large. As long as your oral presentation skills and material are good, your audience will not become irritated or 'switch off'.

- Do have a backup of your slides – try to have them on two USB memory sticks or floppy disks. In the past, one of the authors has been in the situation where a presentation on a USB stick has become corrupted, but fortunately, a backup was always available.
- Once you have produced your slides (and this can take some time as you try to continually improve them), you have to think about your talk. First of all, make sure that you really do know your research and the background to it. It is much better and more interesting for your audience if you address them freely rather than read from a prepared paper.
- Try to anticipate what questions you may be asked – and work out your answers.
- If you have never spoken at a conference before, gain confidence (because oral presentations are all about confidence) by a simple device used by one of the authors. Close your eyes and open a

dictionary at any page, and then pick out a word at random by pointing anywhere on the page. No matter what it is, try to speak on it for five minutes. Even if you do not know what the word means, still speak about it – make something up. The idea is to gain confidence that you can 'think on your feet'.

- Practise your presentation over and over again – initially on your own, and then in front of friends and colleagues, who can help you by critiquing and offering useful suggestions.
- Another tip to help you gain confidence: it is always a good idea to remember that, as regards your research, you will know much more about it than anyone else there, because you are the person who has undertaken the research – nobody else. After all, if your audience did know more than you about your subject and research, then, first, there would have been no need for you to do your research, and secondly, it would be someone from your audience who would be on the podium doing the presentation, not you. If you bear this simple fact in mind, you will be much more confident.
- Finally, as part of your preparation, practise your timing. At conferences there are many presentations to be given and you may be given a fixed time limit (e.g. 20 minutes) – as will everyone else – so timing is crucial. If you run over your allotted time you will be cut off before you have finished or, worse, you will run over your time and the next speaker will not have their full allotted time. Think also of how more nervous you might be if you were kept waiting to give your presentation.
- The other thing about timing is finish your presentation before your allotted time is up – this is to allow for questions from the audience. So, when preparing your presentation and practising it, do allow about five minutes from your 20 minutes for questions. That will leave you about 15 minutes for your actual presentation – not long to get your ideas and research findings across – so you have to avoid waffle.

You have practised your presentation until you can give it in your sleep and the day has arrived when you are scheduled to present your paper. As the day arrives, your nervousness is bound to increase. The authors of this book are both very experienced at presenting at conferences, but still get nervous just beforehand. It is important to relax, otherwise you will not do yourself, or your research, justice.

So, the day has arrived. Check everything beforehand: that your slides work, that you are in the right place for your presentation (large conferences often have simultaneous sessions in more than one room) and that you are appropriately dressed.

When you are standing before your audience, there are some things that you have to be careful to do to enhance your presentation:

- Stand up straight – don't slouch on the lectern (only very experienced presenters can get away with that, even though they shouldn't). You should show your audience respect.
- Speak slowly, loudly and clearly – particularly if you are speaking at an international conference where English may not be the first language of many in your audience. Both authors have attended conferences in which English is not the language of the conference, and it can be very tiring and bewildering to follow what is going on, even if you have a good knowledge of the language being spoken.
- Change the pitch and tone of your voice (difficult if you are reading from a prepared paper) as without this your presentation will be very monotonous and you will lose the audience's interest and attention.
- Try to think of your presentation as a drama and speak as if you are acting in a play – include changes of expression and dramatic pauses (this is where all the practice you did beforehand will come in useful).
- Don't be afraid to make the odd joke or come out with a wry expression – anything to hold the attention of your audience – but not too often, or your research will not gain the respect it deserves. But remember: different nations tend to have their own cultural sense of humour and what may be funny for one country's nationals may not be for nationals of another – or may even be even offensive to them.
- Interact with your audience at all times. If it fits in with your presentation, then have the audience do some work. One of the authors once gave a 1½-hour presentation at an international conference on the 'new genetics and immunodeficiencies' during which, at one point, all the audience became base pairs (parts of genes) and had to jump up and down in sequence to illustrate a very important concept. There was much merriment, but also a crucial and difficult part of the presentation was actively illustrated, and hence understood, by the audience.
- Maintain eye contact with the audience – it helps them, and it also helps you, to include them in the presentation and it makes them more receptive to what you are saying.
- Importantly, demonstrate enthusiasm for your presentation and your research. After all, if you cannot show enthusiasm for the presentation and research, how can you expect your audience to do so?
- Finally, and most importantly, enjoy yourself! Your 20 minutes or so on the podium will pass very quickly, but if you have engendered enthusiasm in your audience, your presentation will not be

forgotten and people will contact you afterwards to find out more about your research and to discuss your presentation.

Scenario 2

You have undertaken the research that consisted of an interview in which you were the interviewee and for which you decided what was to be the subject (refer to scenario 1 in chapter 8 and scenario 2 in chapter 9). You already have the data that you collected and analysed. Now you want to present these data at a conference.

However, for it to be accepted, you need to write an abstract for the conference organisers. Do this using the data that you have collected and analysed, using the format presented above. Try to keep your paper between 250 and 500 words. This will give you some practice in writing abstracts for conference presentations.

Also, if you have access to Microsoft PowerPoint, prepare no more than four slides that will encapsulate your research (use the guidance above to help you). If you do not have access to Power-Point, then list the points that you would have made on no more than four slides.

This will give you practice in writing an abstract for a conference presentation, and also preparing slides for a conference presentation.

Summary

This chapter has shown you how to make the most of your research in terms of making it available to a wide audience, starting with the research report itself. After all, your research is only as good as the dissemination of its findings. If no one knows anything about the research that you did, then really, what was the point of doing it, except possibly for personal satisfaction? In this case you have to ask yourself if your research participants/patients have derived any benefit – in other words, has the issue of beneficence in your research been demonstrated?

References

Albert T. (2009) *Winning the publications game*. Abingdon: Radcliffe Publishing.

Bordage G. (2001) Reasons reviewers reject and accept manuscripts: the strengths and weaknesses in medical education reports. *Academic Medicine* **76**(9): 889–896.

Buzan T. (1993) *The mind map book*. London: BBC Books.

Clarke G. (2000) Writing for publication. *International Journal of Palliative Nursing* **6**(7): 316.

Department of Health (2006a) *Our health our care our say: a new direction for community services*. London: The Stationery Office.

Department of Health (2006b) *The NHS in England: operating framework 2007–08*. London: The Stationery Office.

Department of Health (2008) *Framing the contribution of allied health professionals: delivering high quality healthcare*. London: Department of Health.

Gray D. E. (2004) *Doing research in the real world*. London: Sage.

Houser J. (2008) *Nursing research: reading, using and creating evidence*. Boston, MA: Jones & Bartlett.

Morse J. (2007) Reasons for rejection/reasons for acceptance. *Qualitative Health Research* **17**(9): 1163–1164.

Munhall P. L. & Chenail R. (2008) *Qualitative research proposals and reports: A guide*. (3rd edition). Boston, MA: Jones & Bartlett.

Murray R. (2006) *How to write a thesis*. Maidenhead: Open University Press/ McGraw Hill Education.

Murray R. & Moore S. (2006) *Handbook of academic writing: A fresh approach*. Maidenhead: Open University Press/McGraw Hill Education.

Nelms B. C. (2004) Writing for publication: your obligation ot the profession. *Journal of Paediatric Health Care* **18**: 1–2.

Offredy M., Cleary M. et al. (2008) Improving health and care for patients by redesigning services: the development and implementation of a clinical assessment service in Harrow Primary Care Trust. *Quality in Primary Care* **16**(2): 95–102.

Parahoo K. (2006) *Nursing research: Principles, process and issues*. Basingstoke: Palgrave Macmillan.

Paul R. J. (2002) Is information systems an intellectual subject? *European Journal of Information Systems* **11**: 174–177.

Perneger T. V. and Hudelson P. M. (2004) Writing a research article: advice to beginners. *International Journal for Quality in Health Care* **16**(3): 191–192.

Polit D. F. & Beck C. T. (2008) *Generating and assessing evidence for nursing practice* (8th edition). Philadelphia: Lippincott, Williams & Wilkins.

The Research Proposal: Current Research Issues in Healthcare

Introduction

At last, you have finished your research proposal, but before we complete this book, we want to introduce you to some of the current research issues that we are experiencing in healthcare research. Healthcare research has come a long way in recent years, as have healthcare and medicine themselves. This is all to the good, and it has certainly increased the quality of care we can offer our patients/clients. However, these advances have brought some problems and controversies in their wake. This chapter introduces and discusses just a few of them.

There are several issues that give cause for concern regarding health research. These include:

- The ethics of undertaking research using human subjects.
- The ethics of undertaking research using vulnerable human subjects.
- The ethics of undertaking research using embryos.
- The ethics of undertaking research using animal subjects.
- The availability of funding.
- The origins and provenance of funding.
- Vested interests regarding the funding, process and reporting of research.
- The politicisation of research.
- The implementation of research findings.

These issues are discussed and explored in this chapter, but a quick glance at the list above shows that ethics is a major contributor to them all.

We started this book by looking at what we mean by 'research', and to discuss it briefly in this final chapter neatly 'bookends' our discussion of how to prepare a research proposal. So let us begin by looking again at what we mean by research. It is a word that is banded about, but do you know what it means and what it involves? Whenever you are not sure what a word means, it is always a good idea to consult a dictionary. According to the *Shorter Oxford English Dictionary* (2007) 'research' has many meanings, but the ones that are relevant to our research are:

- 'The action or an instance of searching carefully for a specified thing or person.'
- 'A search or investigation undertaken to discover facts and new conclusions by the critical study of a subject or by a course of scientific enquiry.'
- 'Systematic investigation into, and study of, materials, sources, etc. to establish facts, collate information, etc.; formal postgraduate study or investigation; surveying of opinions or background information relevant to a project, etc.'

These definitions make a good starting point for thinking about and doing research. There are, however, issues that arise concerning the difference between research and clinical audit. This is may be confusing for nurses because they are often required to carry out clinical audits in the course of their work and may think that they are undertaking research. In reality, the two processes are quite distinct and should not be confused.

Research is designed to provide new knowledge, the findings ensuing from it possibly being of value to others who are in a similar situation (generalisability). At the same time, these findings, and the whole process of the research project which produced them, are available for critical scrutiny and are accessible to everyone.

Clinical audit, on the other hand, is concerned with the process of identifying the quality (or its lack) in an existing service (or one that is being planned) to see if it meets defined standards for that care or treatment. In addition, clinical audit can be used to identify methods and processes that may improve the care or treatment that has been audited.

The whole subject of what research is and what clinical audit is and their differences is discussed much more fully in chapter 1, but is reprised here because of issues based on the need for ethical approval for research and clinical audit. If a project, particularly one involving humans, is classed as research, then it will almost certainly require approval from an ethics committee (see chapter 6) as all research involving patients and staff must have ethical approval before it can be carried out. Normally clinical audits do not require ethical approval from a committee, although sometimes clinical audits do have an ethical element, in which case they will require approval from a research ethics committee.

How do you know whether your clinical audit project (or indeed your research project) requires ethical approval? For all research, and for clinical audit if you are uncertain as to whether you require ethical approval, contact your local R&D office for advice; alternatively, you can contact the chair or administrator of your local ethics committee.

Finally, we need to consider why we do research. Why is it important? The Canadian Paediatric Society (2008: 707) states that 'health research is a moral duty because it is the foundation for evidence-based care by all health care practitioners'. In Australia, the National Health and Medical Research Council (2000: xi) puts the case for the importance of research – albeit more practically – when it states:

> 'health and medical research provides the base that enables improvements in health care and clinical medicine, as well as the development of a high quality health care workforce. Advances arising from health and medical research in Australia will continue to benefit the Australian community, in terms of improved treatment and health care services, while also delivering a more cost-effective service.'

In addition, healthcare research is important because:

- It aids nurses – as well as doctors and other healthcare workers – to improve the care that they give to their patients/clients.
- It increases knowledge – but to what end? There is a gap between knowledge for its own sake and knowledge for practical means.

Perhaps for more selfish reasons, research in general also is important because:

- It confers prestige on the researchers (and the institute in which they are situated).
- It is necessary for certain academic qualifications and for careers.
- It is interesting
- It is fun!

So, without further ado, let us look at the issues mentioned at the beginning of this chapter.

Ethics

The subject of ethics in research is discussed more fully in chapter 6. In this section we explore some of the ethical dilemmas that healthcare researchers face on a day-to-day basis. These are:

- The ethics of undertaking research using human subjects.
- The ethics of undertaking research using vulnerable human subjects.
- The ethics of undertaking research using embryos.
- The ethics of undertaking research using animals.

The ethics of research using human subjects

The National Health and Medical Research Council report states that 'Contemporary ethical dilemmas in the field of research on humans are many and complex' (2006: 57). It acknowledges that these dilemmas have existed for a long time and can be grouped under the following headings:

- Consent.
- Participant safety.
- Scientific merit.
- Conflict of interest.
- Risk versus benefits.
- Protection of vulnerable people.
- Disclosure of information to participants/families.
- Privacy.
- Confidentiality.

These are covered in chapter 6, so we shall not discuss them again here.

A report by the National Health and Medical Research Council (2006) looks into the complexity of the ethics of undertaking research on human subjects and notes that there are four main factors that contribute to this increasing complexity:

1. Advances that have taken place in medical science, particularly over the past 50 years or so. These advances have opened up new possibilities that were not even thought of previously (e.g. gene replacement therapy, major organ transplants).
2. The increasing breadth, as well as depth, of research on humans. They note that research on humans has extended way beyond drug trials and experimental fields, and into the sort of research that nurses and other non-medical healthcare workers undertake (e.g. in the fields of behaviour, attitudes and psychosocial concerns).
3. The increasing globalisation of research, and the implications of this for local ethics committees regarding the consequences of their decisions in the long term and the management of the research that they have before them and on which they must make a decision to approve or not to approve.
4. The level of specialisation that is required to assess and scrutinise some of the proposed research proposals. This is not only in the sciences, but in disease pathology and other specialties (e.g. sociology, psychology, nursing).

Thus, the increasing complexity of research involving humans, as demonstrated in these four points, gives rise to decision-making about ethics that 'requires either an entirely new approach or an integrated approach of a kind the particular committee has never before confronted' (National Health and Medical Research Council 2006: 58).

The ethics of undertaking research using vulnerable humans

One aspect of research using human beings is, of course, research using vulnerable human beings (see also chapter 6). This section links the previous section (human subjects) with the next (embryos) because embryos are extremely vulnerable (although the argument could be made that they might not be fully human).

Just who is vulnerable when it comes to research? Well, one could argue that everybody who participates in research is vulnerable, because there are often perceived power differences between the researchers and the participants. Some people, however, due to illness, age or limited intellectual capacity, are particularly susceptible and vulnerable (e.g. children). With children, the problem of informed consent is especially acute, as are the physical, intellectual and developmental differences between them as children and the researchers as adults. Research with children, however, just as with research with all types of patients, is recognised as being morally necessary; in other words, it is a moral duty as long as the research is based on ethical principles (Canadian Paediatric Society 2008) and is concerned mainly with:

- **Distributive justice** – making high quality healthcare available to all, including vulnerable children.
- **Beneficence** – providing high quality care which will benefit all.
- **Non-maleficence** – avoiding harmful therapies.

As the Canadian Paediatric Society (2008: 707) states: 'children may be harmed if health care providers do not provide care based on the best available evidence.'

However, there are many more vulnerable groups of patients than just children – for example, people with mental health problems and people with life-limiting illnesses (e.g. cancer, HIV).

In terms of undertaking research with vulnerable people, it has been argued that palliative care is faced with more moral problems than are found in any other areas of healthcare (Randall & Downie 1999). Similarly, it is often argued that palliative care has a specific moral dimension (Janssens et al. 1999, Hermsen & ten Have 2001). Hermsen & ten Have (2001) argue that if this is the case, then palliative care will include moral issues that are intrinsically related to it. With this philosophical and ethical argument in mind, one of the areas in which the ethical dimensions of palliative care come to the fore can be found in all aspects of research in this group of patients. However, unless research is undertaken with these patients then their care will never improve. As both Karim (2000) and Polit & Hungler (1999) strongly point out, it is the vulnerability of patients undergoing palliative care that is a major issue arising out of the sensitivity of actually conducting research with them.

Turning to research involving patients accessing palliative care, Polit & Hungler (1999) point out that conducting research with people who are dying is problematic because of their particular vulnerability as they may be at high risk of unforeseen and unintended side-effects due to their particular circumstances. Consequently, Polit & Hungler (1999) feel that these patients need more protection than is given by the general framework of ethics and ethical research guidelines.

What are these vulnerabilities that have to be taken into consideration by a researcher involved in research studies with patients accessing palliative care and their families? Karim (2000) identifies seven concerns:

1. Patients often experience complex symptoms as well as mental and physical exhaustion and may be quite frail – to put it bluntly, they may not be in any condition to participate in a research study.
2. The research, particularly if it raises potentially painful issues surrounding death, might result in the patients experiencing psychological distress (Aranda 1995).
3. Although willing to take part in the research, patients might find it increasingly difficult to do what is being asked of them – they may well experience cognitive and physical deterioration that could affect their ability to complete questionnaires, self-assessment or quality of life scales, or even to be interviewed. Another problem around the issue of cognitive deterioration raised by Addington-Hall (2002, citing Pereira et al. 1997) is that where patients have evidence of cognitive impairment, this can lead to impaired decision-making capacity, and all that that can imply, particularly in terms of giving informed consent.
4. Patients who have not yet reached the terminal phase of their illness may have other demands on their time (e.g. frequent hospital outpatient appointments, regular moves between home, hospital and hospice) according to their care needs. This may mean that finding time for interviews or to complete questionnaires is tricky.
5. Karim (2000) also mentions that patients who are relatively well may not find it easy or convenient to spend their time filling in questionnaires or taking part in interviews. Family members may resent the patient spending time taking part in a research project because they themselves want to spend time with them. Addington-Hall (2002) points out that many questions have been asked about whether it is ethical to ask patients accessing palliative care to participate in research. This could risk depriving them of energy and time when the time could possibly be better spent allowing them to attend to unfinished business, as well as just being with their family.
6. Patients may be trying to distract themselves from their illness or its symptoms. Involving them in research will make them focus on their illness and dying.

7. Finally, patients may agree to sign the consent form but only because they fear that if they refuse, it may jeopardise with the way their professional carers manage their care. As Karim (2000, citing Randall & Downie 1999) points out, this raises the question of whether any patient participation in health research can ever be voluntary, because there will always be an unspoken fear that by not taking part in the research, the patient may be penalised. This point is supported by Addington-Hall (2002), who argues, as others have, that it is unethical to ask patients to participate in research as they may feel coerced, or may be unwilling to give an honest evaluation of the care they receive.

To conclude this section, Lee & Kristjanson (2003) stress that without research, there is a risk that nothing new will be attempted and that there will be a failure to scrutinise how we care for dying people. In addition, they point out that without research to demonstrate and justify the value of palliative care services, palliative care providers may find it increasingly difficult to attract funding.

From a social justice perspective, as Rawls (1971) suggests, all members of the community have an interest in the provision of good healthcare because each member of that community may need healthcare in the future, and some may need access to palliative care. Therefore, each member of the community has an interest in ensuring that good palliative care is available – care that is based on the best evidence provided by ethical research.

Seymour & Ingleton (1999) argue that it is important that we develop models of research for accessing users' views. However, in terms of palliative care, as Seymour & Skilbeck (2002: 219) state: 'this requires striking a fine balance between the ethical duties of providing caring support, nurturing independence and autonomy, and achieving research outcomes that are rigorous while also being accessible and meaningful to users.' Researchers have a responsibility to ensure that their findings will be of value and that the rights of the participants are protected. They should acknowledge and honour the rights of palliative care patients, families and healthcare workers who choose to be involved in their research. It is only through research into the experiences and needs of patients accessing palliative care, and their families, that palliative care researchers and clinicians can better understand the needs of the community and improve the quality of the care they provide (Lee & Kristjanson 2003).

Thus, the point is well made that research needs to be undertaken with people who are vulnerable – indeed, one could say that it must be undertaken – if we are to improve our care of them.

The ethics of undertaking research using embryos

This remains highly contentious in research circles, as well as among scientists, politicians, people with strong religious convictions, humanists and the general public. Where you fall in this debate depends on your background, convictions and what you believe embryos to be. Do you believe that an embryo is a person? If so, then you will be governed by your views on the ethics of undertaking research with human subjects.

What is an embryo? Embryo research takes place in the very early days of the development of the embryo when it is basically a bundle of cells with few of the characteristics that we associate with a human being both anatomically and physiologically – it is simply a fertilised human egg. On the other hand, this fertilised egg does have the capacity to become a person if left to develop. While still an embryo, though, it has no brain, no consciousness or self-awareness, and certainly no neurological function that will allow it to feel pain or experience emotion. An embryo is consequently not capable of suffering physically or emotionally.

So, our thoughts and decisions are guided by how we view the embryo at this early stage – a bundle of cells with no feelings, or a potential human being with all that that implies. This is the moral dilemma that we, and those either supportive of or against embryo research, have to wrestle with.

There is a further moral dimension to this problem: what do we intend to do with these embryos – i.e. what is the research for? Embryo research is a vital part of our research into the treatment and cure of many catastrophic medical conditions (e.g. Parkinson's disease, Alzheimer's disease, diabetes, spinal cord injury) (Sandel 2004). Are we denying the right to health, and even life, of others if we refuse to allow research to take place using human embryos? To counteract that, we need to look at the discussion on research ethics (chapter 6) and the difference between maleficence and beneficence. Certainly for the embryo, research on it is harmful as it always dies, and certainly there is no benefit that accrues to it from the research.

This debate requires a whole chapter, if not a whole book, to do it justice, but to move on we shall briefly summarise both sides of the argument, which is linked to the belief of when life begins.

- **Against embryo research:** all conclusions against embryo research are based on the fundamental belief that a human life begins at conception – when the egg is fertilised. Consequently, the embryo is seen as a human being, with all the rights accruing to being human, at the very moment of conception. As far as those against embryo research are concerned, any experiments that put the embryo at risk are not only unlawful they are morally abhorrent – the ethical equivalent of medical experiments on unwilling or uninformed victims (after all, the embryo cannot give permission for the experiment). In addition, although the research could lead to new, life-saving treatments, the embryo is eventually killed or, at the very least, is put at great risk. Is this justified, no matter what the potential benefits to mankind in general may be? In other words, the ends should not justify the means.

- **For embryo research:** all conclusions for embryo research by those who support it are based on the belief that life does not commence at the moment of conception. That gives rise only to a 'potential' human being, as opposed to an actual one. Where you stand on the potentiality of being a human being compared to actually being one determines whether you are in one camp in this argument or in another. Consequently, people who are for research using embryos tend (but not necessarily always) to advocate that an embryo becomes a human being when:
  - the foetus (not an embryo – they are two separate stages of development pre-birth) comes to resemble a human being rather than a bundle of cells;
  - the foetus is at a viable stage in development (i.e. could live independently outside the uterus);
  - the foetus has developed neurologically to the point that it can experience pain and self-awareness;
  - at birth, or at some other stage of the pregnancy that is as yet not defined

(www.embryoresearch.co.uk).

You have probably detected a flaw in this, namely, that all these are at different stages in a pregnancy – even the moment of the birth of a viable baby can have a span of four months (from 23/24 weeks to over 40 weeks), so how can you pinpoint the moment that life begins?

Another point is that people who believe in research using embryos still have strict guidelines to which they have to adhere, namely:

- Such research is only justifiable if there is the reasonable possibility of medical knowledge and human life being enhanced by the research.

To sum up, there are two very strong, controversial and fundamentally opposing views (and many shades of belief within them) concerning embryo research, and there are very good moral, ethical and scientific viewpoints for both arguments. As we stated at the beginning of this section, where you stand depends on many factors, but it is important to debate this for it brings into focus a very important, if not vital, question – what is a human being, and when do we become one?

The ethics of undertaking research using animals

Although this is not something that nurses, or even doctors, do, you need to be aware that there are concerns expressed by many in society about the use of animals in medical research, particularly the use of primates. However, many of the arguments for and against the use of animals in health research are the same as those for embryos being used in research. If you think about it, you will easily see the similarities, although many would argue that animals exist for us to use. After all, we eat them, but we do not eat human embryos. Similarly we use their skins or pelts for clothing, but not the skins of human embryos. Consequently, many are not concerned about the use of animals for human health research and do not give it much thought, but it is important to look at all the moral imperatives in research that impinge on our health.

Funding issues

The availability of funding

Funding for research is always a matter of concern for any researcher. You may have an excellent research proposal, but without funding it is virtually worthless. Depending on the type and size of your research project, funding may be required for:

- paying staff undertaking the research;
- the infrastructure required to undertake the research (e.g. a laboratory, a place to interview participants);
- computing systems to allow for data analysis;
- stationery and tape recorders/video recorders for interviews;
- payment for transcribers of interviews, statisticians for data analysis, interpreters if interviewees speak a language you do not;
- travelling expenses, postage and other stationery

(Clifford 2004).

There are other requirements for funding according to the type of research that you intend to carry out and the resources already available. So, where does funding come from and how do you access it?

Funding from research can come from many different institutions and organisations. For a long time, funding for healthcare research (particularly for clinical healthcare research) has been available in the main teaching hospital centres in the UK. Since 1948, the National Health Service (NHS), recognising that there is a link between healthcare, education and training, and research, established an early research base for medicine (and doctors) in general (nurses and others working in the NHS at that time were deemed not to be able to do research). Since then, the government has helped to fund medical research through the Medical Research Council (MRC), established in 1913.

The introduction of the Regional Health Authorities in the 1960s led to the funding of small-scale research projects – mainly for consultants and research scholarships for junior doctors. At the same time, a number of medical charities (e.g. cancer charities), as well as hospital trust funds, have funded a lot of R&D studies (Shaw & Clifford 2004). It was the more recent development of R&D centres in individual hospitals that led to the current interest in funding nursing and other healthcare professionals' research, and the realisation that such research was as important as medical research because the overall care of patients was so important and necessary for the restoration of good health, and that it was important to have a well-educated and knowledgeable nursing and healthcare professional workforce that could look at the nursing (and other) care that was being given to patients in a scientific and systematic way. Nurses and other healthcare professionals have an important role to play in healthcare research because their direct input into nursing (and other) care makes them ideal for contributing to healthcare research.

But where are you going to get your funding from to allow you to commence and complete your research? What you must bear in mind is that only about one in seven bids for research funding are successful, as there is a lot of competition. As a consequence, you need to spend a great deal of time and effort on your research proposal to make it 'stand out from the crowd' and be the one in seven that is chosen.

There are many organisations and institutions to which you can apply for funding, including:

- government organisations;
- universities;
- hospitals;
- diseases charities (e.g. cancer, heart disease, diabetes);
- general charities (e.g. Nuffield);
- pharmaceutical companies;
- other companies and industries (e.g. the tobacco industry);
- nurses' organisations;
- other healthcare professional organisations.

Of particular help and importance in the UK for nurses is the Royal College of Nursing (RCN), which works in partnership with RDFunding (part of the National Institute for Health Research – NIHR) to help you find sources of research funding. Other potential sources can be obtained from the RCN website:

> http://www.rcn.org.uk/development/researchanddevelopment/funding/funding_opportunities.

When you come to write a proposal for your own research, good luck with your search, and application, for funding.

The origins and provenance of funding

As a researcher, you will be keen to obtain funding from just about anywhere.

However, there are pitfalls to be aware of. Some important questions to ask are these:

- Where does the money come from?
- Is the source morally sound or is it linked to various medical, physical, social, psychological, employment or environmental abuses?
- What do I have to do to receive this funding?
- What is expected of me?
- Will I be free to report on my research without interference? (See below.)
- What levels of access to data will I be able to obtain, e.g. will anything be 'out of bounds'?
- How secure is my funding?

Your research will need to be seen to be free, unbiased and uncontaminated by outside interests; therefore, the provenance of your funding has to be uncontroversial.

Vested interests regarding the process and the reporting of research

These are often linked to where you get the funding for your research from (see above). But it also concerns the motives of the participants in your research study, and is often a problem with the use of volunteer sampling (see chapter 7).

If your funding comes from a pharmaceutical company, for example, how much control will they have over your research as regards methodology, data and report? If, as may be likely, your research is linked to their product, will you be free to criticise it if necessary? Will you be able to select your own sample without interference? Will they make all their data available to you?

The same applies to other industries. A notable example is the tobacco industry. This gives rise to much discussion as to the ethical, legal and policy issues around its funding of scientific research for 'tobacco companies have an interest in portraying a positive corporate image. Scientists have an interest in unrestricted grants. The tobacco control community has raised – and continues to raise – concerns about tobacco industry funding of external research' (Society for Research on Nicotine and Tobacco 2003: 1). Indeed, the SRNT (2003: 1–2) points out that 'several U.S. schools of public health and organisations that fund tobacco-related science have instituted formal policies restricting their faculty from accepting tobacco industry funds.'

But it does not just apply to drug companies and other commercial interests. Special interest groups and charities may also have a vested interest in 'managing' your research. Or they may be concerned with your findings and put pressure on you not to release your final report if it is not to their liking.

Even colleagues can have a vested interest in your not writing anything that may show them or their work in a poor light. This may not be for their own sake, but they may want a favourable report to obtain funding for their own work. That can put a lot of self-applied pressure, as well as pressure from colleagues, on you, because you may feel that the future of your department is at risk.

However, if you are going to undertake research, you need to be strong and objective about your results, otherwise it is better not to start the research in the first place. All research has to be honest, truthful and objective, no matter what the circumstances.

The politicisation of research

This is linked to the previous section, but is a particular worry. The worry is not so much about interference by political interests (although this does go on), but rather the use to which your research – and your findings in particular – may be put by anyone with a political agenda to fulfil. This is discussed in chapter 8 (data collection) on the way in which statistics can be manipulated to fulfil a particular agenda (it is illustrated with some excellent quotes). This happens all the time in every country and now has a new term – 'spin'. There are endless reports of political parties and individual politicians putting a spin on an item of news. This can happen with your research when only the results from your research that favour someone are publicised and others results are put to one side or discounted. Of course, the opposite may also happen.

The media in particular are very good at putting a spin on someone's research results. However, because of their need to sell newspapers (and that means going for the sensational rather than the 'truth') they are often only interested in problems rather than good and positive findings.

The pressures put on researchers by vested interest, politicians and the media are not rare. The author of this chapter has personal experience of some of the pressures and the 'spinning' of results. When publicising your research, these are some of the things that you need to be aware of and neutralise if at all possible.

The implementation of research findings

This final section discusses the importance and practical aspects of implementing your research findings in practice.

Why is it important to implement your research findings? Well, the answer is that it is not always important to do so, it depends very much on:

- the type of research that you have done;
- the results that you have obtained;
- whether or not your findings are suitable for implementation.

Not all research is geared to practical/clinical work, but may be theoretical. In this case, it is meant to increase our knowledge of a certain subject rather than be used in a practical sense. However, it is important for your research findings to be disseminated in print and/or as presentations at conferences (see chapter 10). After all, if you have spent months or even years on your research project, at the very least you want to let others know what you did and what you found.

Secondly, your results may have been inconclusive and therefore not suitable for changing practice. Or they may just simply confirm the status quo. Therefore, implementation of your research results is not an option.

Thirdly, your results may not be suitable for implementation because, for example, they would be too expensive. Alternatively, there may not be the human and material resources to implement them.

A further reason for non-implementation could be that what you are proposing is ethically or morally not right, for example, it may go against the ethos of the unit.

However, assuming that your findings are suitable for implementation, a number of stages need to be gone through as part of this implementation:

- negotiation of access to the organisation;
- identification of a contact person or local change agents within the organisation (e.g. educational, managerial and clinical);
- teaching personnel their roles once the implementation has taken place

(Smith & Masterson 1996).

Taking the first point above – the negotiation of access to the organisation – this does not just mean your being able to gain physical access to a particular unit, or other site, in which you wish to implement your research findings. You also have to persuade the managers and other personnel that your research findings are accurate, valid and unbiased. This requires you to answer questions, and give assurances, as to the methodology, sampling, funding and ethics, and also (and perhaps most importantly) that your findings will help to improve the care that is given in that unit.

The next stage is to do with 'change' theory and includes the identification of relevant change agents in the organisation. This is a crucial stage in the implementation of research findings.

Change is an important part of our lives and of our being. We all need to be able to change things, whether in our professional or our personal lives. We cannot stand still. At the same time, any changes we make need to be well thought out, otherwise they could be a disaster. Consequently, any change that we need to institute needs to be 'managed'.

Managing change has at least two meanings, but only one is relevant to our situation. This is the making of changes in a planned, managed, systematic fashion. The aim here is to implement more effectively new methods and systems within an ongoing organisation. The changes to be managed lie in, and are controlled by, the organisation itself. They are internal changes. However, these internal changes might have been triggered by events from outside the organisation – in our case, by our research findings (Nickols 2004).

You will recall that we need to gain access to the organisation in order to implement our research findings. This is usually someone from management as they are often the 'gatekeepers' for the organisation. Management also has to be able to assess/estimate what impact any change could have on employee behaviour patterns, work processes and motivation (hence the importance of thoroughly briefing them on your research study and findings at the outset). Management must also assess what the employees' reactions are likely to be when confronted by potential changes.

In addition, they will need to be able to devise and introduce a change programme that will provide support as employees go through the process of adapting to change. Before they do this, however, they will need to identify one or more change agents. Change agents are (usually) people from within an organisation who have a thorough grasp of the changes to be made and the rationale for them. In addition, they must support the proposed changes, because their role is to plan the changes (often in cooperation with management) and to 'drive' them until they are in place. Thus, they must have a plan for:

- the implementation of the change;
- dissemination of the change throughout the relevant part of the organisation;
- monitoring the effectiveness of the change;
- making adjustments to the change where this is shown to be necessary.

So, to sum up, a programme of change should:

- describe the change process to all the people involved and explain the reasons why the changes are occurring – this information should be reliable, unbiased, transparent and timely;
- be designed to effectively implement the change whilst remaining within the overall organisational objectives, macro-environmental trends and employee perceptions/feelings;
- provide support to employees as they deal with the change, and wherever possible, involve the employees directly in the change process itself.

Change agents – and you, as the researcher, may well be one of these – usually need a model of change to allow them to make changes in a scientific, rational, orderly and systematic way. There are many models of change, including perhaps the most well known – Lewin's (1951) model (see below). However, we shall begin with a very simple model which is one that most nurses and other healthcare professionals are familiar with – problem-solving.

Problem-solving

This is a very useful framework for thinking about change. In this process/model, managing change is seen as a matter of moving from one state to another – from the problem state to the solved state. Diagnosis or problem analysis is essential – goals are set and achieved at various levels and in different areas or functions. Ends and means are discussed and related to one another. The outcome is a transition from one state to another in a planned, orderly fashion – this is the planned change model (Nickols 2004).

Some people prefer to use the word 'opportunity' rather than 'problem' because of the negative connotations that that word carries. However, from a rational, analytical perspective, a problem is nothing more than a situation requiring action but in which the required action is unknown. Therefore, it is necessary to search for a solution, and this search activity is known as 'problem-solving'. At the heart of change management lies the change problem, and this manifests itself as a:

- What? problem.
- How? problem.
- Why? problem.

The 'What?' problem includes the following questions that you need to ask yourself or your fellow change agents:

- What are we trying to accomplish?
- What changes are necessary?
- What indicators will signal success?
- What standards apply?
- What measures of performance are we trying to affect?
- What skills do I have that will allow me to make this change?

The 'How?' problem' asks:

- How would we do this?
- How do we get the resources?
- How can I find out more about this?
- How can I overcome any research barriers?
- How can I find the time to do this?

The 'Why?' problem asks:

- Why do I want to do this?
- Why do we have to change the way we do things?
- Why do I need to involve other members of the team?
- Why is this important?
- Why don't I just forget it and go and make another cup of tea?

(Nickols 2004).

Kurt Lewin's (1951) model

Although an early model of change, the model developed by Lewin (1951) is still a favourite one, particularly for novice 'changers'. This framework is useful because it allows us to consider a stage-by-stage approach – in other words, 'looking before you leap'.

Lewin describes change as a 'three-stage' process:

- Stage 1 – 'unfreezing', which involves the disposal of the status quo. It is during this stage that others' defence mechanisms have to be overcome or bypassed.
- Stage 2 – 'changing'. This is when the change occurs. This is considered by Lewin to be a period of confusion. During this stage, we are aware that our old ways are being challenged, but we do not have a clear picture of what to replace them with.
- Stage 3 – 'refreezing'. This occurs once the change has been completed. The new changes are becoming embedded and people begin to feel more comfortable with them. In other words, a new status quo is in operation.

The beginning and end point of Lewin's unfreezing–changing–refreezing model is **stability**.

Much of change management theory is based on common sense, and we are certain that if any of you have attempted to make changes in your professional life, then you may well have considered all that we have discussed in this section without actually putting it into a theoretical framework. It may even be possible to use the Nursing Process as a model for your change, although it is not as well structured as Lewin's model. But then again, you can always 'mix and match' and take the best of Lewin's, the best of problem-solving and the best of the Nursing Process in order to develop your own model depending on the change that you are going to discuss.

This brings us to the third point – teaching personnel about their new roles once the implementation has taken place. Obviously, any new processes, cares, therapies or treatments need to be taught to those who will be implementing them. This is where it helps to have a teacher as one of the change agents. However, it is as well to be aware that:

- You may get some resistance from staff to the changes.
- In the worst possible scenario, attempts may be made to sabotage the changes.
- There may be a lack of understanding and some confusion as to why the changes are necessary and what exactly what they are.
- Finding time, money, space and other resources for the teaching sessions may be difficult because of overstretched staff with little free time and a lack of available resources.

However, do not be depressed by this, because you may find:

- Members of staff are eager to learn about these changes and to implement them.
- You will receive full backing from management who will arrange for staff time and other resources to be available to you and the change agents.

Even with the backing of factual evidence (your research findings), it may be hard to change entrenched practices (Hunt 1984). However, good research and its implementation are important litmus tests of professional status (Thomas 1987). If we fail to create professionalism based partly on research and clinical evidence, then nursing as an art and a science will be lost (Bassett 1993). As Carter (1996) states:

> 'critical evaluation of research findings in terms of their implications for practice and a readiness to change existing practices where appropriate should go some way to addressing these concerns (loss of nursing professionalism) and will be to the benefit of nurses as well as the patients that they care for.'

Summary

This chapter has looked at several, but by no means all, the issues associated with the process and implementation of research. These have included the ethics of undertaking research, particularly on vulnerable participants, and problems associated with funding, politicisation and vested interests. The aim has been to stimulate you to think about the issues and pitfalls associated with research, not necessarily just for when you do some research yourself but also for when you read research studies and research papers. Hopefully, you will now be able to analyse them in terms of these issues, rather than just accepting them.

We have also looked at the implementation of research findings – why they are important, how you start to implement them and the problems you may encounter when you attempt to implement your findings and to make changes in practice.

This chapter will close by asking a question – is implementation of research findings the *raison d'être* (the whole reason) for undertaking research? You may not have been able to answer it before, but as we are reaching the end of this book and the web program hopefully you will now be able to answer it and give reasons for your answer.

Activity

Think of something that you would like to change about your own practice or the practice within your specialty, and then attempt these activities:

- Make two lists – one of the reasons for changing the practice the other of the reasons for keeping it. Compare them and see which are the stronger and more compelling reasons.
- Now think about who would be your change agents, and why.
- Finally, write a plan of how you would systematically go about changing the practice – what steps you would take and why. What resources would you need and – in your own practice – what would be the likelihood of your being able to access these resources?

By now you will have an idea of just what is involved in systematically making a change in practice.

References

Addington-Hall I. (2002) Researcher sensitivities to palliative care patients. *European Journal of Cancer Care* **11**: 220–224.

Aranda S. (1995) Conducting research with the dying: ethical considerations and experience. *International Journal of Palliative Nursing* **1**(1): 41–47.

Bassett C. C. (1993) Role of the nurse teacher as a researcher. *British Journal of Nursing* **2**(8): 911–918.

Canadian Paediatric Society (2008) Ethical issues in health research in children. *Paediatric Child Health* **13**(8): 707–712.

Carter D. (1996) Barriers to the implementation of research findings in practice. *Nurse Researcher* **4**(2): 30–40.

Clifford C. (2004) Introduction. In G. Clifford & J. Clark (Eds.) *Getting research into practice*. Edinburgh: Churchill Livingstone.

Hermsen M. A. & ten Have H. A. M. J. (2001) Moral problems in palliative journals. *Palliative Medicine* **15**: 425–431.

Hunt, J. (1984) Why don't we use these findings? *Nursing Mirror* **158**(8): 29.

Janssens M. J. P. A., Zylicz Z. & ten Have H. A. M. J. (1999) Articulating the concept of palliative care: philosophical and theological perspectives. *Journal of Palliative Care* **15**(2): 38–44.

Karim K. (2000) Conducting research involving palliative patients. *Nursing Standard* **15**(2): 34–36.

Lee S. & Kristjanson L. (2003) Human research ethics committees: issues in palliative care research. *International Journal of Palliative Nursing* **9**(1): 13–18.

Lewin K. (1951) *Field theory in social science.* New York: Harper & Row.

National Health and Medical Research Council (2000) *Health and medical research strategic review: Implementation of the government's response – final report.* Canberra: Commonwealth of Australia.

National Health and Medical Research Council (2006) *Challenging ethical issues in contemporary research on human beings.* Canberra: Australian Government.

Nickols F. (2004) *Change management 101: A primer.* http://home.att.net/~nickols/change.htm.

Pereira J., Hanson J. & Bruera E. (1997) The frequency and clinical course of cognitive impairment in patients with terminal cancer. *Cancer* **79**: 835–842.

Polit D. F. & Hungler B. P. (1999) *Nursing research principles and methods.* Philadelphia: Lippincott.

Randall F. & Downie R. S. (1999) *Palliative care ethics. A good companion* (2nd edition). Oxford: Oxford University Press.

Rawls J. (1971) *A Theory of Justice.* Oxford: Oxford University Press.

Sandel M. J. (2004) Embryo ethics – the moral logic of stem-cell research. *New England Journal of Medicine* **351**(3): 207–209.

Seymour J. E. & Ingleton C. (1999) Ethical issues in qualitative research at the end of life. *International Journal of Palliative Nursing* **5**(2): 65–73.

Seymour J. & Skilbeck J. (2002) Ethical considerations in researching user views. *European Journal of Cancer Care* **11**: 21.

Shaw H. & Clifford C. (2004) Research in healthcare: establishing a national research and development programme. In G. Clifford & J. Clark (Eds.) *Getting research into P practice.* Edinburgh: Churchill Livingstone.

Shorter Oxford English Dictionary (6th edition 2007) Oxford: Oxford University Press.

Smith P. & Masterson A. S. (1996) Promoting the dissemination and implementation of research findings. *Nurse Researcher* **4**(2): 15–29.

Society for Research on Nicotine and Tobacco (2003) *Tobacco funding and scientific research workshop: Ethical, legal and policy issues – summary* http://cancercontrol.cancer.gov/tcrb/tfms.pdf.

Stem Cell Research UK, *What is embryo research?* www.embryoresearch.co.uk.

Thomas E. A. (1987) Pre-operative fasting – a question of routine? *Nursing Times* **83**(49): 46–47.

Index

Note: page numbers in *italics* refer to figures and tables.